Achieving True Wellness *in a* World *of* HEALTH LIES

Unveiling the Confusion, Myths, and Deceptions Keeping You from Lasting Health

DR. JACKIE McKOOL

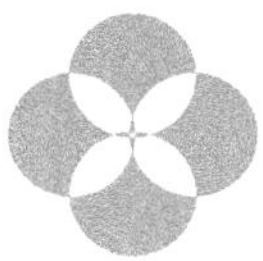

ENDORSEMENTS

"Each one of us takes a journey into increased health awareness. I believe as you read Jackie's journey you will be inspired and will pick up additional clues as to steps you can take to improve the quality of your life and be able to celebrate your golden years with a body that still works and can enjoy and celebrate life. So, dig in and see what you can discover.

I fully agree with Dr. Jackie that vibrant health includes spirit, soul, and body. All three must be given attention. Anyone which you ignore will be at your own expense. So, buckle up for the ride and learn from Jackie's story."

Mark Virkler
President – Communion With God Ministries &
Christian Leadership University
Author of *"4 Keys to Hearing God's Voice"*
Co-Author of *"Restoring Healthcare as a Ministry"*

"Seeing Dr. Jackie McKool grow into this new chapter of her life was my privilege. I watched her learn and grow from the Internal Disorders Diplomat program into a broader scope, wholistic understanding of health and wellness, and implement these principles into her practice as a board-certified chiropractic internist. This book shares many of those insights she learned through the DABCI program."

Virginia Kessinger,
Wife of the late Dr. Jack Kessinger, ProHealth Seminars

"I have known Dr. Jackie McKool for nearly two decades. There are few people who have walked and overcome life adversities on a path of spiritual awakening as Dr. McKool has done. Wisdom and truths can quickly be found reading and following what she has to offer, will save everyone a lot of time searching through the noise, deceptions about health, wholeness and life!"

Dr. Frank King
Owner, President
King Bio Homeopathics, and Dr. King's Carolina Bison Farms
Author of *"The Healing Revolution: Eight Essentials to Awaken Abundant Life, Naturally "*

"This inspiring book combines Jackie's personal story of redemption with practical guidance on holistic wellness, rooted in faith and grace. It emphasizes the healing power of non-inflammatory foods, nutrition, and mindset to help readers transform their health. With simple steps and spiritual encouragement, it offers a sustainable path to renewed vitality and purpose."

Tricia Cooper
Health and Wellness Coach

Minister
Author of *"Honey Badger, Hoot, and Honey Bunny"*

"When it comes to health and wellness, it seems that there is so much to learn in so little time. The trick is, will the information be presented in such a way that anyone can understand and implement it with *confidence*? Dr. McKool's book has turned what I thought I knew about health completely upside down. This book explains major health issues many of us in the U.S. face that are caused by stress, inflammation, and poor lifestyle choices; and offers ways to *implement* change to end the vicious cycle of dis-ease in our lives. As a licensed massage and bodywork therapist, helping my clients to implement a more wholistic approach to their wellness is a crucial part of my profession. *"Achieving True Wellness in a World of Health Lies"* has been a foundational resource for myself, my family, and the clients I have the privilege to care for. If you are seeking, here it is. If you are knocking, the door is open."

Josie Lee Varela Whisnant
Licensed Massage and Bodywork Therapist
Breaking Bread Bodyworks, LLC

"If taken to heart, this book can change your life for the better. Jackie offers sound advice coupled with tips that truly work to help you in your "wholistic" journey. I love how she brings our whole being—physical, mental, emotional, and spiritual--into the becoming healthy process, not just food and calories. Emotional trauma can cause us to overeat sweets or other processed foods, falsely thinking they will make us feel better.

Jackie does a wonderful job not only explaining the truth and lies about food but also about a wholistic lifestyle. With all I've learned, I'm ready to implement many of her suggestions, starting with drinking more filtered water. If sick and tired of being sick and tired, I hope you'll join me in the endeavor to achieve wholistic health."

Norma Poore
Award-winning Author; speaker;
and managing editor for Almost an Author website

"I have had the privilege of knowing Dr. McKool for several years and she practices what she teaches. She has personally given me guidance during my own recent health crisis. Her book, "Achieving True Wellness in a World of Health Lies" is a wealth of common-sense knowledge on a wholistic view that the medical field does not always teach."

Karen Clemons
Course Attendee & Student of
"Achieving True Wellness in a World of Health Lies"

"Dr. McKool's passion for wholistic health runs deep, as does her faith in God. Her testimony in this book is nothing short of inspiring."

Tory Haas
Entrepreneur, Speaker, Writer

Achieving True Wellness *in a* World *of* HEALTH LIES

Unveiling the Confusion, Myths, and Deceptions Keeping You from Lasting Health

DR. JACKIE McKOOL

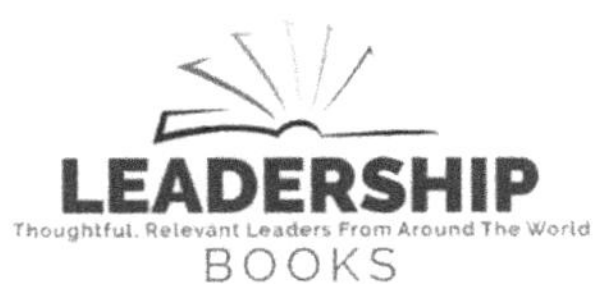

Most Leadership Books products are available at special quantity discounts for bulk purchases for sales promotions, premiums, fund-raising and educational needs. For details visit our website at www.leadershipbooks.com

Achieving True Wellness in a World of Health Lies, by Dr. Jackie McKool
Published by Leadership Books ***or***
Published by Pharresia, an imprint of Leadership Books.
Las Vegas, Nevada & New York, NY

International Standard Book Number:
Paperback:
Hardcopy:
E-Book ISBN:

Printed in the United States of America

A Note from the Author

Thank you for picking up this second edition. While the heart and message of this book remain the same as the first edition, you'll notice a few updates designed to improve your reading experience. The chapters have been thoughtfully reordered for better flow and clarity, and the book has been given a new title and cover design to more accurately reflect its message and purpose.

These changes were made in response to valuable reader feedback and my own continued growth and insight since the original release. I pray this edition serves you even more deeply on your journey toward true wellness and wholeness.

In grace and truth,

Dr. Jackie McKool

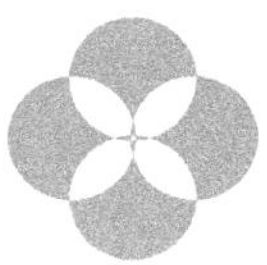

Dedication

I dedicate this book to my mom, JoAnne McKool, who was always my biggest cheerleader when it came to my writings.

Love you, Mom—miss your voice and words of encouragement.

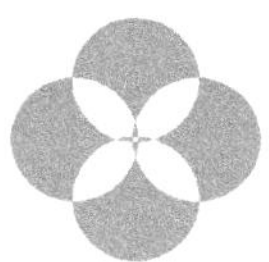

Acknowledgments

My acknowledgments really are more of a prayer. A prayer of gratitude and appreciation for so many. Starting chronologically, I'd like to thank Jesus Christ for delivering me from my addictions and putting my feet on a new path—a wholistic path. And for planting that seed of passion in me to share the truths He was showing me, with others.

I'm thankful for my first chiropractor, Dr. Ken Sable for encouraging me to embark on a career in the chiropractic field; and my chiropractor in Charleston, Dr. Bruce Gwinnup for introducing me to the chiropractic internist diplomate program. Both of whom played a big part in influencing my life on this wellness journey. For Dr. Jack Kessinger, of whom so many truths that I share in this book I learned from him. I pray that the passion he sowed into me through his many hours of teaching will not go unnoticed by him as he rallies with the others in that Great Cloud of Witnesses—you are right Dr. Jack, "it's not tough to be number one" when pursuing the truth about wellness.

I am grateful for all of the many patients, clients, customers, students, social media followers, family, friends, colleagues, neighbors, and even total strangers that I've had the joy to interact with over the years by discussing, debating, and sharing with you the truth about wellness. Your own personal health journey and questions have continued to inspire me and give me fodder for this book. Thank you to the many family members and friends who have been patiently encouraging me to finally write this book I have been talking about for too many years, and for your many, many prayers for me. Truthfully, I was afraid God was getting ready to say to me "move over Moses, I'm bringing Aaron in to do what I have called you to do!" I know beyond a shadow of a doubt He has assigned me to fulfill this task for Him, and I am grateful He didn't give up on me and allowed me to fulfill this assignment for Him!

A special thanks to my dear spiritual mentor and friend, Anna Raymond, for funding the tuition for me to attend my first writer's conference many moons ago, I pray that the seeds you sowed into me will now bear much fruit. A special thank you also goes out to Ron Elmore as well. As my business coach, one of the primary recommendations you gave me the first day we met was that I needed a book, not knowing that it had been a passion burning in my heart for years. You encouraged me that a book was vital to enhance the other two gifts I have that go hand in hand with this book, the other components of my calling—speaking and teaching.

I'm grateful for the opportunity I had to not only serve by teaching, but to learn from women who were walking out their recovery from addiction. This opened up a whole new awareness of the importance of wholistic health to a unique and valuable population of our communities. I love you ladies and pray that at least a few seeds you allowed me to sow into your lives have come to fruition for you.

There are so many others that I met in the early stages of the first edition of this book who helped walk me through a new journey of not just creating my first book, but welcoming me into the writer's community in general; to each and every one I want to say "thank you." Some of you I met at the Carolina Christian Writer's Conference, others of you I met as fellow Christian authors who were more than willing to guide me through the process. And lastly, I am grateful for God's divine appointments–with all of you, but also with my editor, Mari Florence with Leadership Books. Mari "gets it"–she personally has an appreciation for the message of true health, which made our working together so much easier! Thank you, Mari!

My closing prayer for this book is that many, many lives—adults as well as children—are restored back to good health, and even kept from falling down a disease path, so that God is glorified through them as they walk out into all that God has called them to be and do, healthy and whole. Amen.

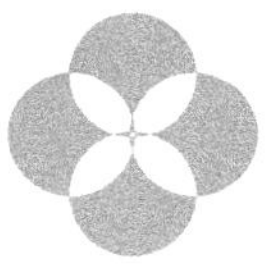

Table of Contents

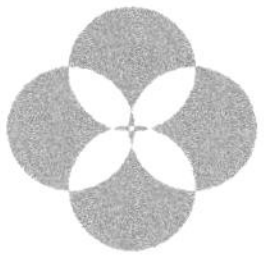

Foreword

We live in a world with varying opinions on effectively managing diagnoses and various health challenges.

Unfortunately, I have witnessed a growing population of people mentally "paralyzed" and rendered powerless when attempting to choose a path to address their illnesses.

In addition, the public has been fed a truckload of falsehoods from sincere and, in most cases, well-intentioned physicians attempting to help their patients.

All medical disciplines follow guidelines called Standards of Care. Medical specialty boards within each specialty set the knowledge and competency expectations through their certification process, which influences treatment decisions by defining best practices within that field.

Does the Standard of Care or Best Practices within a specific medical discipline truly address the root of a patient's health issue? Does it consistently achieve optimal clinical outcomes?

The answer is NO!

Working with thousands of patients throughout my 20 years practicing functional medicine, I have seen the most challenging cases with most patients simply confused and disheartened about their lack of improvement for their unresolved physical sufferings.

Again, almost all traditional physicians have good intentions to help their patients get well, but most must follow their training and have only a few tools in their toolbox.

These tools almost always consist of drugs and surgery, which traditional doctors incorporate as mainstays while managing their patients.

Some provide some level of dietary counseling, but it is simply lacking in any meaningful application without a full understanding of nutrition and lifestyle management.

According to most studies, medical doctors in the United States typically receive less than 20 hours of nutrition education throughout their 4 years of medical school, which is significantly inadequate compared to the importance of nutrition in overall health.

All the above brings me to Dr. Jackie McKool's beautiful book *Achieving True Wellness in a World of Health Lies.*

This gem of a book had me taking notes on each page, enthusiastic about what I was going to learn next.

The book reads like a novel, sharing personal insights that make the reader get to know Dr. McKool, the author who has lived what she writes about.

Her book will grip you and have you nodding in acceptance with her outlook.

As I am one not to stand in the corner about my Christian walk, I appreciate her openness and transparency; she gives all the credit to God for answering a prayer of purpose in her life.

I am proud to be part of her Christian walk and to help her share the good news about true wellness.

As Dr. Jackie states, *I know with all my heart and soul that God's purpose for my life is to share these truths with others like you so you can also live a life of purpose—one that is healthy, whole, and free of sickness and disease.*

Achieving True Wellness in a World of Health Lies is a roadmap—or better yet a blueprint—to achieving true wellness.

It is *not* a typical book that gives you a checklist for achieving health.

Her book does provide crucial, detailed information, but she provides a needed twist not commonly seen in most health-related books.

She provides her unique perspective on the meaning and interpretation of why we get sick and what keeps us sick. She calls it semantics.

For some readers, Dr. McKool's book will serve as a paradigm shift their thinking about health.

However, her book is not for those simply looking for a quick fix. Individuals seeking such a solution will best be served by the traditional medical approach of drugs and surgery.

On the other hand, if you like, thousands of my patients are sick and tired of being sick and tired. Achieving *True Wellness in a*

World of Health Lies will be a breath of fresh air and will help you in new and unexpected ways.

Her elegant but insightful book's pure truth on health is almost never addressed by conventional medicine.

If you are like the millions of people ready to restore their health, Dr. McKool's book will be a true blessing for you and your family and friends. The strategies outlined in this book will take commitment, but truly obtaining ultimate health and well-being will be worth more than anything money can buy.

Remember: even if you have a vast amount of wealth, it holds little value if you lack good health. Your health is more important than money and should be prioritized. True health really is true freedom.

Learn to embrace true health by reading and studying Dr. McKool's *Achieving True Wellness in a World of Health Lies.*

It will change the trajectory of your health in ways you never imagined.

Enjoy your new health journey by embracing and applying all that Dr. McKool will share with you.

Sincerely,

Ronald Grisanti D.C., DIANM, D.A.C.B.N., M.S., CFMP
Board Certified Chiropractic Orthopedist
Diplomate, International Academy of Neuromusculoskeletal Medicine
Diplomate, American Clinical Board of Nutrition
Master of Science in Nutritional Science from University of Bridgeport
Certified Functional Medicine Practitioner
Founder and Medical Director of Functional Medicine University
Website: www.FunctionalMedicineUniversity.com

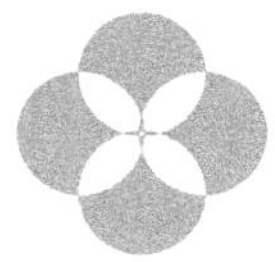

Preface

Imagine a World Without Sickness and Disease...

> "'For I know the plans I have for you," declares the Lord, "plans to prosper you and not to harm you, plans to give you hope and a future." (Jeremiah 29:11 NIV)

Come follow me on a little journey.

Start by relaxing. Close your eyes, quiet your mind, and breathe slowly and deeply. Now, let your imagination stretch as far as you like. Imagine a world without sickness or disease, without physical or emotional pain. What would it look like? What would it feel like? No cancer or chemotherapy, no depression or anxiety, no disabilities, no hospitals—not even children's hospitals.

But even more than that, imagine always feeling great. Sleeping soundly, having more energy than you know what to do with from sunrise to sunset, looking fantastic, thinking clearly, mastering self-control and discipline. Even your desires and dreams become reality because now you can function at your optimum potential.

How perfect would all this be? It sounds like it would be "... on Earth as it is in Heaven" (Matthew 6:10 NIV). Well, I have good news: all this can be a reality—or at least far better than it currently is.

This picture isn't just for a few; it's for everyone. Thousands, if not millions, are already living this way. You can be a part of this group of people who live long, healthy lives free of pain, sickness, and disease. It is truly possible if you have the tools to make it happen.

But first, you must believe it's possible and commit to change no matter the cost—not just financially but also in terms of time and effort. The challenge is not the cost itself; it's shifting from a *desire* to a *commitment* that prevents people from moving forward. If you commit for the long haul, your world can be a lot freer from pain, sickness, and disease. It takes lots of hard work, but it is so worth it!

When the seed of purpose was planted in my heart back in March 1996, it felt as though the blinders had been removed from my eyes. For the first time, I could see beyond my next hangover and recognize endless possibilities—not just for myself but for those around me. If only they, too, could see it.

It all started with the newfound certainty that I had a purpose in life and that life was to be lived *wholistically*.

As a new Christian seeking God's path, I clearly heard Him speak to my heart. He told me to enroll in chiropractic school at nearly 40 years old, but I sensed all along that chiropractic was not to be my ultimate destination, merely a stepping stone toward my greater purpose.

After I graduated and set up my practice, the real learning began—not just in honing my chiropractor skills but also in firsthand experiences of wholistic health through the unique needs of my patients. Each case offered insight into the requirements for complete healing.

I continued refining my wholistic approach by growing in my spiritual walk with God. I underwent emotional and spiritual healing myself then learned to minister to others in the same way. I sought ways to improve my mental resilience and maintain a healthy balance in my life—not just professionally but personally. I worked toward financial freedom, managed my commitments, and pursued goals that aligned with my ultimate purpose.

I became my own test subject whenever possible, experimenting with new lab tests, supplements, foods, exercise regimes, and more. I wanted to share my insights with patients to help them lead healthier lives, to be a pioneer for those within my sphere of influence.

After 10 years of practice, I found myself in Western North Carolina, managing a small health food store at the foothills of the Appalachian Mountains. This may have been my favorite job yet. I had the tremendous opportunity to educate customers every day as they sought ways to improve their health beyond mere disease management. I was in my sweet spot. As they learned from me, I learned from them. I remained in this industry for 3 years before moving on to the next phase of my wholistic journey.

I then became the development director for a women's ministry that worked with women in addiction recovery. This experience deepened my understanding of wholistic healing for a new population. I saw firsthand how recovery could be dramatically improved by addressing the *mental*, *emotional*, *physical*, and *spiritual* aspects from a natural, wholistic approach.

During these transitions, my parents passed away within 18 months of each other. Upon their passing, they blessed my brothers and me financially. One day, I woke up debt free, seeing my 10-year goal finally come to fruition. More importantly, it allowed me to step into the *peak fulfillment* of my purpose—the one God had bestowed upon me 26 years prior: to *educate*, *encourage*, and *empower* others along their wholistic healing journey through speaking, teaching, and writing.

This book and its accompanying course are tools that help fulfill my purpose and passion—to see others set free and guide them onto a path of wholistic healing, just as God did for me 30 years ago.

My prayer is that you, too, will glean greater insight into how you might walk fully in all God is calling you to be and do—healthy and whole.

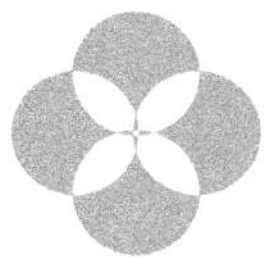

Introduction

On March 6, 1996, I rolled into bed drunk shortly before 7:00 a.m. A couple hours later, I was calling in sick at work, telling myself I was done with drinking. I had officially hit rock bottom.

I'd like to say I was finally disgusted and ashamed enough that I quit drinking. I was, but in truth, it was Jesus Christ who delivered me from this stronghold on my life. Although this time was no different than the dozens of other times I'd told myself the same things, it was because of Him alone that I made different choices.

Over the past 30 years, I have come to realize that "apart from Him, I can do nothing" (John 5:15)—the very first scripture I ever memorized. I also came to realize that "I can do all things through Christ who strengthens me" (Philippians 4:13). This verse carried me through chiropractic school at more than 40 years old.

This book is a result of my own journey of uncovering deceptions and discovering the truths about wholistic health and wellness. My spelling of wholistic with a "w" is intentional. Because my focus is on the *whole* person, I prefer *wholistic*. I know with all my heart and soul that God's purpose for my life is to share these truths with others like you so you can also live a life of purpose—one that is healthy, whole, and free of sickness and disease.

I was raised in a middle-class family in Johnstown, Pennsylvania, a small rural town in the southwestern part of the state. Growing up in the 1960s and 1970s with three younger brothers, my life was very typical for that era. I attended Catholic grade school and graduated from public high school. Our neighborhood was full of kids, and I spent much of my time outdoors year round.

For 8 years, I walked about a mile to grade school, and when I attended high school—5 miles away—I either rode my bike, took the bus, or, from age 16 on, drove myself in my bright yellow 1970 Ford Maverick. My mother, like many in that era, became excited by the convenience of new packaged and processed foods hitting the market. With four rambunctious children (and one more 11 years later), she did whatever she could to carve out an extra hour in the day.

At age 22, I left Johnstown and moved to the Eastern Shore of Maryland for a couple of years before heading to Southern Maryland, near Washington, D.C. It was there that Jesus took hold of my life and set my feet on a new path—a path of wholistic health and wellness. On March 6, 1996, He delivered me, at age 36, from a 20-year addiction to alcohol, the bar life, and everything that goes along with that kind of living.

In that moment, He planted a passion in me—not only to pursue greater health for myself but to share these truths with others. At the time, I envisioned storming into barrooms, yanking people off their barstools, and proclaiming with great excitement, "Do you realize there is a whole other world out there? Come follow me! Step out of this dark (literally and spiritually), dingy place into the light!"

My journey accelerated quickly, and before I knew it, I was heading to chiropractic school at Sherman College in Spartanburg, South Carolina, at almost 40 years old. After graduation, I set up a chiropractic practice in Charleston, South Carolina, for 10 years and pursued a postdoctoral degree in internal disorders. While Sherman College laid the foundation for my chiropractic philosophy, my additional 2 years of postgraduate study provided deeper clarity on wholistic health and wellness. In 2007, I earned a board certification as a chiropractic internist, becoming a Diplomat of the American Board of Chiropractic Internists (DABCI).

As a new Christian, I became aware of the deceptions I had been taught—about everything from evolution to false religions to nutrition myths like "fat is bad for you." I had believed these lies to be truth. This realization planted a seed of hunger in my heart for the real truth—to know truth in Jesus Christ, to speak truth in obedience to His commands, and to reveal truth to others.

One of my pet peeves is to hear people, including myself, tell "white lies". I try very hard not to lie by omission or avoidance. Am I perfect with this? Of course not. But I don't like any kind of lie or deception—especially when it comes from me.

As I built my chiropractic practice, I saw firsthand how patients were being deceived about true health and wellness. This deception prevented them from achieving and maintaining optimum health and healing. This hurt my heart, and it still does. Few things pain me more than seeing people suffer because they are unknowingly deceived—especially about their health.

Being from the North, I tend to speak my mind, sometimes when I shouldn't. More times than I care to admit, I find myself opening my mouth and inserting my foot. I have a deep desire to expose deception and reveal the truth, but Ecclesiastes 3:7b says, "…there is a time to be silent, and a time to speak." Learning when to be silent has been a long, hard lesson for me. This is why I needed to write this book—so I can speak truth in love and so you can choose to accept it, or not, when you are ready to hear it.

You have a *choice* about how to take care of your health. Without knowing you have a choice, you might continue down the path of sickness and disease, thinking you are doing the best you can when, in reality, you are not because you have been unknowingly deceived.

Most importantly, *you* have a unique divine purpose for being alive. Without you, we all suffer—your family, your friends, even strangers. You matter to people you may never meet as well as others who influence you directly in ways you may never know—for better or worse. If illness prevents you from fulfilling your purpose (or worse—if you leave this earth too soon), where does that leave the rest of us who need you?

This book is for you and for all of us.

This is *not* just another "eat your veggies and exercise" book. Yes, those are important, and we'll discuss them. But this is about much more than that. This is about wholistic health—mental, emotional, physical, and spiritual. I won't be telling you to follow a certain diet; I'll share something bigger.

This book is about semantics—those subtle lies that keep us sick. It's about how we become sick without even realizing it. I will share the true meaning of wholistic health through little anatomy lessons on some very vital organs and systems of the body that, if addressed wholistically, can go a long way toward a much healthier life. When you have a true understanding and appreciation of how your body works, you will be *empowered* to make it work for you rather than against you.

I'll also expose long-held deceptions that prevent us from achieving optimum health and healing. Finally, I will provide tools to help you on your healing journey. Ultimately, my prayer is that this book will encourage you and give you many "aha" moments.

Your health *is* in your control. That is *empowering*, and it is *freedom*!

Once you have finished reading this book, don't keep this information to yourself. Truths are meant to be shared. By sharing this book, you can help bring others out of the darkness of deception.

After all, we each have a purpose, and we need one another.

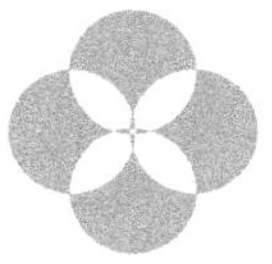

SECTION 1

Clearing the Muddied Waters: A Paradigm Shift toward True Wellness

I'm all about truth. Shortly after becoming a new Christian, the scales began falling from my eyes, revealing truths that I had not seen before. This awakening ignited a deeper hunger and thirst for God's truth. It also hurt my heart to see others walking in the same darkness in which I had once been trapped. As a result, truth has become one of my core values.

When I first delved into functional medicine through my practice, I worked hard to educate my patients on the *truth* about wellness. However, I quickly realized that, while they *thought* they understood wellness, we were often communicating on two parallel paths. The miscommunication stemmed largely from semantics, where, as in most deceptions, "a little leaven spoils the bread."

I love the New Living Translations version of Galatians 5:9: "This false teaching is like a little yeast that spreads through the whole batch of dough!" That's exactly what I witnessed with my patients. They longed for better health and genuinely believed they were making the right choices yet saw no real progress.

It was during this time that I first developed my *Truth About Wellness* health talks. These talks evolved into newspaper columns, blog posts, and ultimately, this book—along with its accompanying workbook and online course. Truth is vital to every one of us achieving optimum health and function.

In this first section, I will address some common semantics that can hinder our ability to achieve true wellness. Additionally, we will explore each area of the wholistic health framework, breaking down an approach to each component that is rarely, if ever, addressed by conventional medicine.

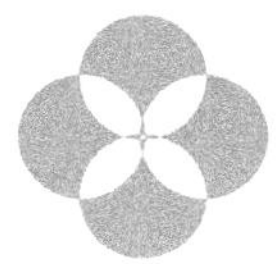

CHAPTER 1

The Truth about Where Health Comes From

> *"You made all the delicate, inner parts of my body and knit me together in my mother's womb. Thank you for making me so wonderfully complex! Your workmanship is marvelous—how well I know it. You watched me as I was being formed in utter seclusion, as I was woven together in the dark of the womb. You saw me before I was born. Every day of my life was recorded in your book. Every moment was laid out before a single day had passed."*
>
> *—Psalm 139:13-16 NLT*

My dad was a private pilot. He never flew anywhere without his maps. He used them to set the instruments in his plane, and those coordinates guided him to his destination. But if those coordinates were off by even just one degree, and he flew far enough, he could end up in Alaska instead of Florida! The same is true for your health. What are you aiming for? Are your coordinates set toward true wellness, or are they unknowingly aligned with disease management?

You might think you feel pretty good. Maybe you have no diagnosed diseases, or maybe you take one small medication for blood pressure or cholesterol. Does that mean your health is truly optimal? Why bother making changes if your life already seems fine?

There's always room for improvement. More importantly, what about the fate of the next generation? The people you influence—your children, family, and community—may not end up as healthy as you. And if you believe their sickness and disease won't affect you, think again. We are all connected.

The absolute *first* thing you must realize is that you have a unique, divine purpose for being here on earth. *You* are the *only* one who can fulfill your calling. Until you recognize and accept this responsibility, your motivation to achieve optimum health will miss the mark.

If you don't care that you may die at the age of 50, 60, or even 70 from a preventable disease, (and yes, seventy to 80 percent of chronic degenerative diseases, including autoimmune diseases and cancers, are self-induced), you are neglecting your unique responsibility—not just to yourself but to the rest of the world as well. When you are not well, we all suffer. This is not just a "feel-good" or "positive-thinking" statement; it's the truth.

The *second* most important realization is that you must make a paradigm shift in your thinking. There is an entire world of people who approach their health in a completely different and far more effective way. The main difference is the *objective*: they focus on identifying the root cause of the problem and restoring the body's natural ability to heal rather than just managing disease. This is the essence of the wholistic approach.

The *third* critical mindset shift is understanding that your health is within your control. It truly, truly is. Once you have embraced this truth, you are on your way to a better, healthier life.

Health Comes from Above, Down, Inside, Out

In chiropractic school, we had a saying: "Health comes from above, down, inside, out." This means that health comes from God (i.e., above), and from within—the integrity of the internal environment (i.e., inside our bodies), and outward. This is the truth.

We have been taught to believe in a problematic "outward–inward" mentality. We assume that something external—germs, fate, genetics—"get" us sick. We shift the blame, thinking we have nothing to do with our health conditions. This is where our coordinates have veered off course.

Ever since the germ theory was introduced by Louis Pasteur in the late 1800s, our medical system has followed the wrong map. It has led us to believe that disease comes from outside influences alone instead of recognizing that internal health plays a crucial role.

Will I Ever Be Healthy Again?

Have you been diagnosed with a chronic, degenerative disease like diabetes, high cholesterol, high blood pressure, heart disease, irritable bowel syndrome, colitis, hypothyroidism, or obesity? Or maybe an autoimmune condition like lupus, multiple sclerosis, rheumatoid arthritis, or celiac disease? Have you been told that you are doomed with this disease for the rest of your life, dependent on medication forever?

These things can be reversed! You are *not* doomed to suffer for the rest of your life. Your health is within your control—far more than you realize.

The first step in reversing disease is changing your mindset about the true nature of health. When you begin to align your coordinates with true wellness rather than disease management, you will be amazed at what is possible.

The journey to optimal health and healing starts now.

The Two Main Objectives to True Health

The first step toward true health is deciding which path you want to take. Do you want to manage your disease through drugs and surgery, following the conventional model of disease management (i.e., the germ theory model)? This may seem like the easier route. Or do you want to pursue true health and wellness, uncovering the root cause of illness and restoring your body to optimal function using natural methods—the wholistic health approach (i.e., above, down, inside, out)?

Before making your decision too quickly, let me share a very classic example of how two different approaches to the same issue can lead to totally different results.

A Personal Health Journey

In January 2022, I contracted COVID-19. By April, I was experiencing severe mid-thoracic back pain that radiated down the back of my right arm. Naturally, I called my chiropractor. The relief was temporary. After my second visit in as many days, she took my blood pressure; it was high. I was astonished, as I'd never had high blood pressure before.

A friend of mine—an extremely fit athlete who had completed triathlons and mountain biking races —had recently suffered a massive stroke. With that in mind, I took my symptoms seriously. Without that knowledge, I would have brushed it off as a simple spine misalignment.

When the pain returned, I went to Urgent Care. I had only been there once, years earlier, when I broke my leg backpacking. I asked them to rule out a heart attack. An EKG came back normal, but my blood pressure was still high. The doctor's only recommendation? Blood pressure medication.

The physician I had never seen before proceeded to give me standard advice: lose weight (ha!), don't eat salt (ha again! we'll get to that later), exercise, and lower my stress. He obviously had no clue that he was preaching to the choir! I told him I would not take the blood pressure medicine, and his parting words of advice were, "*Well, then, get yourself a blood pressure cuff and keep an eye on your blood pressure.*" He also informed me that most people die of heart attacks at 2:00 a.m.—well, that was comforting!

The Conventional versus the Wholistic Approach

Many people would have simply taken the prescription, unaware that getting to the root cause was even an option. Had I followed the conventional path, I likely would have been on blood pressure medications—plural—for life. Instead, I chose a wholistic approach.

I *did* take the doctor's suggestion to monitor my blood pressure, and it continued to be high. So, I sought out a functional medicine doctor. His approach was different from the start. He asked for any past bloodwork and reviewed lab tests I had previously dismissed. What we found was concerning: my red blood cells (RBCs), hemoglobin, hematocrit, and platelets had been gradually increasing throughout the past 2 years. That was the first problem.

He also understood COVID-19 could reactivate dormant infections such as the Epstein–Barr virus and various herpes viruses. After ruling out cardiovascular concerns (which COVID-19 can also trigger), he ordered antibody tests. The results revealed COVID-19 antibodies and elevated Epstein–Barr antibody virus markers. I remember having mononucleosis as a kid—Epstein-Barr is its underlying virus. COVID-19 had reactivated it.

Now I had a subclinical infection—I was not contagious and had no acute symptoms, but the virus was still affecting my body. Research has shown that COVID-19 reactivates dormant viruses and can either trigger or worsen autoimmune conditions.

Digging Deeper: Autoimmune Markers and the Body's Stress Response

We ran an advanced autoimmune panel, testing seven different autoimmune markers. The results showed elevated levels in several areas, indicating a potential autoimmune process in motion. Though I wasn't experiencing classic autoimmune symptoms, I did have high blood pressure, episodic vertigo, nail bed pain, and mild fatigue—things that could have been dismissed as simple effects of a busy lifestyle.

How does all this relate to high blood pressure? Inflammation.

When stress and inflammation are present in the body—whether due to infections, toxins, or other factors—the adrenal glands respond. One function of the adrenal glands is signaling the kidneys to regulate fluid levels and blood pressure. This cascade of stress and inflammation was the root cause of my blood pressure spike.

The Path to Healing

Instead of merely treating the symptom (i.e., high blood pressure) with medication, we addressed the root causes—infection and inflammation. The treatment plan included:

- A noninflammatory diet
- Targeted exercise
- A natural supplement protocol to support immune function
- Other wholistic lifestyle changes, which I will discuss later.

By targeting the root cause, I shifted away from disease management and moved toward true health restoration

The Critical Choice: Managing Symptoms or Restoring Health

Had I chosen the more conventional approach, my high blood pressure would have been managed with medication, but the root cause would never have been uncovered or addressed. Over time, my autoimmune markers could have progressed into full-blown autoimmune disease, leading to additional medications for new symptoms. The cycle would have continued indefinitely. Instead, by addressing the root cause, I stopped the disease process before it could escalate. That is the difference between conventional and wholistic health.

Choosing Your Path

Once you decide on your approach, you need to equip yourself with the right knowledge, resources, and healthcare practitioners (whether traditional or natural) who align with your chosen path.

If you want to restore your body to health using natural, wholistic approaches, keep reading—this book is for you! But first, you will need to shift your paradigm surrounding the true meaning of health and wellness. Let's explore the word *paradigm.*

> ***par·a·digm:*** noun *ˈper-ə-ˌdīm, ˈpa-rə-* also *-ˌdim*\\ *: a model or pattern for something that may be copied: a theory or a group of ideas about how something should be done, made, or thought about.*[1]

As you read this book, I encourage you to set aside what you *think* you know about health and wellness. I'm not asking you to forget anything; once you finish, you will want to compare your previous beliefs with what you have learned to make the best choices for yourself.

For now, approach this journey with an open mind—as if you know nothing about health and wellness. Are you ready to explore a new path to true healing?

Begin Here

First, take an assessment of your overall health—mental (e.g., time management, budgeting, career, goal setting, life purpose), emotional, physical, and spiritual. These four aspects form the four quadrants

---

1 https://www.npr.org/sections/13.7/2016/07/18/486487713/what-is-a-paradigm-shift-anyway

of the health pie. To uncover the *root cause* of any health issue, you must determine *which quadrant* holds the underlying problem.

For example, if you constantly feel tired but only get 5 hours of sleep per night due to juggling two jobs, raising four children, and attending night classes at the community college, the root cause likely falls within the mental quadrant. You are burning the candle at both ends! Your exhaustion doesn't call for more coffee, energy drinks, or pills—it calls for a reassessment of your priorities.

Now, let's drill down a little more. Within the physical quadrant, five key elements are essential for achieving and maintaining optimum health:

1. Rest
2. Water
3. Exercise
4. Good nutrition (i.e., nutrient-dense foods in, toxic foods out)
5. Good nerve supply (more about this in a little bit)

Each of these components must be restored, maintained, and kept in good balance. I will discuss them in greater detail in chapters 4 and 5.

These are the foundational steps toward restoring health naturally. If you commit to these principles, you will see marked results. I am excited for you to embark on this journey. Remember, true healing requires dedication—it won't be easy, but it will be worth it. It is FREEDOM.

Take heart: good health *is* within your control. You are not doomed to live with your current disease or potential diagnosis for the rest of your life.

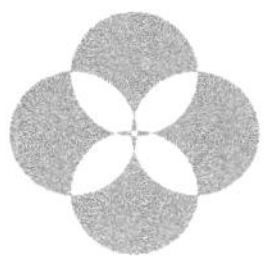

CHAPTER 2

A Paradigm Shift: What Wellness Is Not

"Truth springs from the earth, and righteousness looks down from heaven."

—Psalm 85:11 NLT

When I first started my chiropractic practice in Charleston, I was full of optimism—the kind that only a brand-new practitioner possesses. I was eager to share my knowledge and believed my patients would hang on every word I said about improving their health.

I quickly realized that, while my patients *thought* they were taking natural approaches to health by simply visiting my practice, they were still operating within a disease-management mindset. It was like trying to fit a round peg into a square hole. This disconnect led to frustration—for them and for me.

The Quick-Fix Mentality

We have been conditioned to believe that our health is in the hands of others. Many people have an arms-length approach: *If the doctor says we're healthy, we must be. If the doctor sees something irregular, we must need medication.*

Over time, this system leads to an endless cycle of increasing prescriptions. One or two medications turn into five or six. Eventually, the goal of true wellness becomes a distant dream. But it doesn't have to be that way.

Would you accept a quick fix in other areas of your life and expect lasting results? Probably not. So why do we accept it when it comes to our health?

The Truth about the Magic Pill

I worked in the natural products industry for about 3 years, primarily managing health food stores. During that time, I would have conversations like this every day:

Customer: *"What do you have for headaches, insomnia, energy, etc.?"*

Me: *"I don't know since I don't know what's causing your headaches, insomnia, energy, etc."*

The customer would then look at me like I had two heads! They wanted a wholistic practitioner to engage in the disease management dance with them. That's not what I do.

It's like being at a barn dance and being asked to do the rhumba—it just doesn't fit!

We are so brainwashed with quick-fix thinking that we look for a "magic pill" even when we want to take a natural approach. It doesn't work that way.

Sometimes we reach for processed foods labeled "natural" on the package (which is nothing more than the manufacturer's billboard), thinking that means we're eating healthy. Deep down, we know that is not true wellness.

The Root Cause of Fatigue and Low Energy

When patients and customers used to tell me they were fatigued, lacked energy, or had no libido, my first thought was adrenal fatigue—their adrenal glands were either overworked or already depleted.

Many times, I could smell cigarette smoke on them. I would ask the million-dollar question, *"Do you drink soda?"* Almost always, the answer was *yes*.

I often had conversations with people asking for weight loss advice, citing Dr. Oz. My immediate thought? *Here we go again—the magic pill question*! While Dr. Oz may provide good advice, people tend to latch onto the quick-fix solutions.

I'd ask, *"Do you smoke? Do you drink soda? Do you get enough sleep?"*

The answer was almost always:

Yes (to smoking).

Yes (to soda).

No (to sleep).

Common-Sense Health Truths

Another frequent scenario: Someone seeking an energy boost. When I'd ask about their sleep, they'd say, "*No, I don't sleep well.*" My response? "*Getting more sleep is the answer to your energy problem.*"

Yet they still wanted the magic pill.

Women would ask, "*What do you have for hot flashes?*" When I would start explaining dietary and lifestyle changes that could help, they'd get frustrated because they wanted a quick fix.

There is no magic pill, nor is there even one magic food.

The Common Denominator: Inflammation

In 99 percent of these cases, the underlying issue was inflammation. The more you minimize stress and inflammation, the greater health you will achieve—it's as simple as that.

Some of the primary root causes of inflammation include:

- Lack of sleep
- Inflammatory diet
- Dehydration
- Lack of exercise
- Poor nerve supply

These are a few potential physical causes as well as mental, emotional, and spiritual factors. We will dive deeper into all this as we move through the book.

Wellness Is Not Detecting a Disease Earlier and Starting You on Medications Earlier!

I can't tell you how many times I've had people tell me that they just went to the doctor and were assured that everything was fine. This leads patients to believe that they are healthy, yet they stand before me struggling with all kinds of symptoms and unresolved health issues.

These patients know something is wrong; otherwise, they wouldn't seek help. They feel lousy. They want to improve their health but have been so conditioned to trust the quick-fix approach that it's often difficult to persuade them to see things differently—even when their previous methods have clearly failed.

The Difference between Treating Symptoms and Identifying Root Causes

Discovering the root cause of the body's imbalance may take a little more sleuthing than many people are accustomed to dedicating to their health. While wholistic health practitioners use some of the same diagnostic tools as traditional medicine (e.g., blood work), wholistic practitioners interpret results and prioritize markers much differently.

To visualize this concept, imagine a straight line drawn across a page horizontally. The far-left end of the line would represent 100-percent health, and the far-right end would represent 99-percent disease (100-percent disease would indicate death). This is the *spectrum of health*.

SPECTRUM OF HEALTH

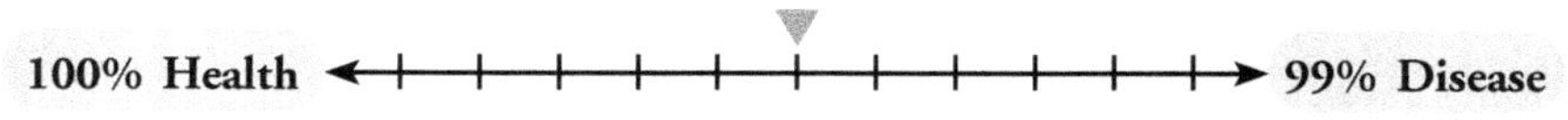

100% Health ◄—+—+—+—+—+—+—+—+—+—+—+—► **99% Disease**

Conventional medicine focuses on the disease end of the spectrum when analyzing blood work. If the numbers are high, you are considered "diseased" and prescribed medication or a medical procedure is recommended. If your results fall within a standard range, you're deemed "fine," meaning no further action is necessary. However, if you are approaching the high or low threshold and a medication exists to address your markers, you may be given a *pre*diagnosis (e.g., a prediabetic prescription) and told "everything is good."

This approach implies that you are either diseased (i.e., at the right end of the spectrum) or healthy (i.e., at the left end of the spectrum), completely overlooking the vast middle ground where most people actually fall. No one is 100 percent perfect, and we are not all diseased, so where are you on this spectrum?

The goal of wholistic health is to gather as much information as possible, including case history, physical exams, consultations, blood work, and specialized testing, to determine where *you* currently stand on the spectrum of health. From there, the objective is to restore your body to its optimal state and move you toward true health (i.e., the left end of the spectrum).

Our bodies are always in motion. We are either moving toward disease or moving toward wellness. Which direction are you heading?

Here is another example of how people are led to believe that detecting a disease earlier is equivalent to wellness.

In April 2022, I developed a kidney stone—the culprit of the pain I mentioned in chapter 1. I have no doubt it was related to

COVID-19, as I had tested positive for the virus earlier that year. Surprisingly—and fortunately—the 9mm stone passed on its own, and I didn't feel a thing (can you say "Thank You, Jesus?"!)

At my follow-up appointment 6 weeks later, the urologist ordered yet another X-ray to confirm the stone was gone. Then, he scheduled me for yet another X-ray a year later to check for potential new stones.

If I develop another kidney stone, I assure you—I will know. I don't need unnecessary radiation exposure to confirm it. Radiation causes cancer, so how is this considered prevention?

This is the false promise of preventative healthcare. Annual screenings like mammograms, prostate exams, and colorectal tests are commonly labeled as preventative measures, but this is a misnomer.

You could get a screening every single day of your life, and it would never prevent anything.

A screening might identify a patient's cancer sooner, but it wouldn't stop the cancer from developing in the first place. This is the equivalent of being put on a road of false hope in a car that doesn't exist.

Worse, it leads people to believe that they don't have to change their diet or lifestyle. As long as they get their annual screenings, they assume they won't get cancer. But *this* is not wellness.

There is nothing wrong with undergoing screenings to keep an eye on your health, but don't fool yourself into thinking they are preventing disease. Prevention is in your daily choices—not in the test result.

Wellness Is Not Taking Natural Supplements for Your Symptoms

If you've taken the first step toward moving away from conventional thinking and searching for a more natural approach, you are truly moving in the right direction! But now, I encourage you to take the next step and shift away from *linear thinking.*

Linear thinking is the conventional medical mindset:

- *Symptom here?*
- *Pain there?*
- *Take this.*
- *Problem solved.*
- *End of path.*

This approach—whether it involves drugs or natural supplements—addresses the symptom instead of the root cause. While natural supplements are a far better choice than pharmaceuticals, using them to mask symptoms will still lead you down the wrong path.

While the symptoms may belong to the physical piece of your whole health pie, their root cause could originate in one of the other three pieces. Simply taking a supplement to remove the symptom is not the solution—it is just a Band-Aid.

Only when you uncover the truth and identify the root cause can you proceed with a truly natural approach.

The Right Way to Use Supplements

I use and recommend nutraceuticals (i.e., professional-grade supplements) for two purposes:

1. To bridge nutritional gaps in even the healthiest diets.

Even when eating well, we often lack certain nutrients. Almost everyone can benefit from foundational supplements, including:

- A high-quality multivitamin and mineral
- Essential fatty acids (EFAs)—particularly omega-3s, though we also need omega-6s and omega-9s in the right quality, quantity, and ratio.
- A good probiotic to enhance the gut's good bacterial flora
- A digestive enzyme to support digestion
- Vitamin D and magnesium—two of the most common deficiencies, yet both are critical for overall health

2. To heal and repair out-of-balance organs or systems

    - Ideally, these supplements should be temporary (i.e., used only while healing takes place)
    - Once the body restores balance, the patient should be weaned off them
    - This only works if you've also changed the behaviors and lifestyle habits that caused the initial problem; otherwise, you're just throwing money away on supplements.

Getting to the Root Cause

What is the root cause of your symptoms?

Don't just replace pharmaceuticals with natural supplements and call it wellness. If you're only masking symptoms—even with natural products—you're missing the bigger picture.

Later in this book, I'll discuss quality supplements and the different types of support your body truly needs to heal.

Wellness Is Not a Shortcut

"If it sounds too good to be true, it probably is!"

No matter how often we hear or say those words, we continue falling for the same old sales pitches—especially when it comes to our health.

We are a quick-fix society that wants to believe there's an easy solution to our problems.

I can't tell you how many times I have been asked about the latest fad or magic potion being sold by discount department stores for weight loss or disease reversal. I'm always surprised that rational people invest their hope in these products.

Are people that desperate to avoid good old-fashioned hard work and discipline? Because that is precisely what it takes to restore your health.

There is no shortcut.

There is no magic pill, potion, shot, surgery, or food that will do the work for you.

If there were, wouldn't we all be healthy and thin by now?

The fact is, good health takes time, commitment, and effort. Only *you* can do it for *you*.

Most people lack the patience to restore their health. We live in a microwave society—one that expects instant results without effort. But the microwave mentality doesn't just fail to cure disease—it causes disease.

Wellness Is Not Easy

> *"For the time will come when people will not tolerate sound doctrine and accurate instruction [that challenges them with God's Truth];but wanting to have their ears tickled [with something pleasing], they will accumulate for themselves [many] teachers [one after another, chosen] to satisfy their own desires and to support the errors they hold . . ."*
>
> —2 Timothy 4:3 AMP

If you haven't figured it out by now, my north star—the source of all truth—is the Bible. This verse from 2 Timothy truly demonstrates the consequences of looking for the easy way out in life—including in our health.

When we step off the path of truth and onto the path of lies, deception, and shortcuts, it never ends well.

When we choose ease over discipline, we start down a slippery slope that almost certainly leads to:

1. A waste of time and money
2. A detriment to our health

An anonymous writer said, "*What comes easy won't last long, and what lasts long won't come easy.*" Wellness takes work. It takes effort. It takes commitment. I told you I would speak the truth!

Insurance Companies Should Not Pay for Wellness

Several years ago, I attended an insurance renewal meeting at my workplace. The agent announced our premiums would increase slightly the following year.

When I asked why, he explained the "we" (i.e., the workforce) had drawn on the group policy multiple times throughout the past year.

But this "we" did not include *me.*

I had never used my medical insurance despite paying into it for years.

Meanwhile, my coworkers ran to the doctor frequently because they chose *not* to take responsibility for their health. That's exactly what's happening in our country today.

Our so-called healthcare model is costing us billions of dollars every year. We all pay for it through (1) higher insurance premiums—even if we never use them, (2) lost revenue for employers when workers take sick days, (3) lower salaries because employers are forced to spend money on insurance instead, and (4) higher taxes to fund government-subsidized benefits.

Worst of all, most of this sickness and disease is preventable—yet we all pay the price. Many people hope changes in policy will spare them the cost of our healthcare system. For example, when the Affordable Care Act (ACA) (i.e., Obamacare) removed preexisting condition exclusions, many thought they were getting a free ride. But make no mistake—nothing is free.

A Better Insurance Model: Rewarding Health Instead of Sickness

Let's go back to the basics for a moment. When I first started driving at 16 years old, my insurance was more than my mom's because I was a higher risk. That makes sense, right? And guess what? For the first 20 years of my driving history, I was probably in a car accident every other year. Most of the time, it was my fault. So, if you're an insurance company, would you assume I was a high-risk driver? Would you raise my rates accordingly?

I haven't been in an accident in two decades (thank you, Jesus!). My insurance company actually rewarded me with a rebate for being a good driver. That too makes sense too, doesn't it?

So here is my question: Why doesn't medical insurance work the same way? If most diseases are preventable (which they are), then why aren't people who take responsibility for their health rewarded with lower rates? If auto insurance can lower premiums for safe drivers, why can't health insurance do the same for people who:

- Exercise regularly?
- Eat a healthy diet?
- Maintain a healthy weight?
- Avoid smoking and alcohol abuse?

Why not reward people for making good choices?

A Wellness-Based Insurance Model

A better system would:

- Incentivize people to take care of their health.
- Allow for lower premiums for those who make healthy choices.
- Offer coverage for things that prevent disease—like gym memberships, organic food vouchers, quality supplements, and wholistic health coaching.

Best of all, it wouldn't have to replace the current system—it could be an alternative plan. If someone prefers traditional medical insurance, they could keep it. But for those who prioritize wellness, a less expensive, wellness-based policy would give them the option to pay less and take control of their health.

Taking Personal Responsibility

Health is not a right—it is a responsibility.

It is *not* your insurance company's job.

It is *not* your employer's job.

It is *not* the government's job.

It is *your* job.

Should insurance companies be regulated to prevent excessive charges? Probably, especially when executives from Blue Cross and Blue Shield of North Carolina received compensation packages totaling more than $9 million in 2020—even after a net income drop from $492 million to $260.5 million in 2019 (David Purtell, *Triangle Business Journal*, March 2, 2021).

But even with regulation, true wellness will never come from an insurance policy—it comes from taking ownership of your health.

The choice is yours.

Health Insurance Is a Misnomer—It Is *Still* Medical Insurance

In a September 2009 bulletin, the American Association of Retired Persons (AARP) stated the organization was "*fighting for a solution that improves health care for our members.*"

I wonder if they realize that having health insurance does not improve health care.

Perhaps one day, they will consider something more along the lines of what I proposed earlier—determining the root cause of health issues rather than just managing disease. More and more, I believe that one reason insurance costs are so high is that we are using the wrong terminology.

While it may seem like I am splitting hairs, consider this: if we continually see the word *health* used in the context of conventional medicine—which manages disease but does not restore health—we start thinking it means the same thing.

It doesn't.

In fact, it couldn't be further from the truth.

This is similar to my dad setting the coordinates when piloting his airplane. If we are continually being told that conventional medicine is health, when it is really medical treatment for sickness, we blindly follow the wrong coordinates. We think we are on a path to health, but we are simply managing disease.

Some people believe that if they have "health insurance," they are automatically insured to stay healthy. That false sense of security leads to an even bigger problem: it may cause them to believe they don't need to take responsibility for their health—after all, they have insurance to cover it.

Wellness Is Not Too Expensive

When I was working in a health food store, I had a conversation with a woman who gave me every excuse under the sun for not following my suggestions to start restoring her health.

After she spoke, I ran through what I silently call the ten "yeah, buts."

Whenever someone gives me ten excuses for not making changes—regardless of their dilemma—I know they aren't ready to take responsibility for their health. I surrender silently and move on.

Her final excuse was "I can't afford to eat healthy."

I looked her in the eye and said, "Do you know what doesn't cost one red dime?"

I could see she was ready with another excuse—another "yeah, but."

Instead, she hesitated. She answered, "What?"

I replied, "It doesn't cost one red dime to *not* eat fast food, fried food, packaged and processed foods, and sugars."

With that, she huffed and walked away.

I was only speaking the truth!

Far too often, I hear the same line about healthy eating versus consuming cheap food-like substances: "It's too expensive to eat healthy!"

It is not that healthy food is too expensive—it's that food-like substances are cheap.

Cheap food-like substances (e.g., fast food, fried foods, packaged and processed products, and sugary snacks) have skewed our perception of food pricing. Before understanding how food is—or should be—priced, we should at least be sure the substance being priced is actually food. The average diet today is not made up of food.

What is Food?

Merriam-Webster defines food as "Material consisting essentially of protein, carbohydrate, and fat used in the body of an organism to sustain growth, repair, and vital processes and to furnish energy."

Another definition states, "Food is any substance consumed to provide nutritional support for the body. It is usually of plant or animal origin and contains essential nutrients, such as carbohydrates, fats, proteins, vitamins, or minerals."[2]

Do most of the products on grocery store shelves meet that definition? If you pass fast food, processed snacks, and sugary drinks under a microscope, would they qualify as actual food? Not even close.

So, when someone says it's too expensive to eat healthy, they are really comparing apples to oranges. Perhaps more accurately, they are comparing apples to garbage.

The Truth About "Cheap" Food

The majority of food products people consume today have been highly processed and manufactured to appear like food, but they are not real food.

They are designed to look, smell, and taste like food, but if you strip them down to their core components, they are nothing more than chemically altered, nutrient-deficient substances.

If a substance does not provide nutrients, it does not qualify as food—at least not by any scientific definition. True food contains:

- Vitamins
- Minerals

2 (https://tinyurl.com/y4vd5s7r)

- Good fats
- Proteins
- Complex carbohydrates

Real food supports the body by:

- Sustaining growth
- Repairing damaged cells
- Providing energy
- Preventing disease

So, if the majority of what we eat today does none of these things, why do we spend money on it? Because we've been fooled into believing it's real food.

Final Thought: The Cost of Health versus The Cost of Disease

Before you say health food is too expensive, ask yourself how much it costs to:

- Take a sick day?
- Manage a chronic disease?
- Maintain a supply of multiple medications?
- Lose energy, vitality, and quality of life?

Because that is the real expense. Health is an investment—not an expense. And the best part? Some of the most powerful health choices cost nothing at all. If you want to save money, start by eliminating the things that are actively making you sick.

Nothing is more expensive than sickness.

What Food Is Supposed to Do

Every cell, tissue, organ, and system in your body is fully dependent on the choices you make every day. Your body must use whatever you consume, whether real food with nutritional value or food-like substances that are nutrient depleting and toxic, as the building blocks for your next cells, next tissues, next organs, and next systems.

In other words, the food you eat today is what makes up the *you* of tomorrow.

The nutrients you ingest provide your body with its only source of essential materials.

If you had a choice, where would you place your priorities when selecting a home for your family? To what extent would you go to ensure it was safe, comfortable, and secure?

Most people will even take out a loan to buy the best home they can. Why don't we apply the same level of care and investment to our bodies?

We can replace a house if we need to, but we only get one body—the one God entrusted to us.

Are you starting to see the truth?

It is not too expensive to eat healthy. It's just cheap to eat food-like substances.

The True Cost of Food-Like Substances

Packaged and processed foods are not real food—they are food-like substances.

Food manufacturers can mass-produce these products at a low cost and high profit. They package and market them to you with carefully designed labels, making you believe they are healthy choices.

Are these cheap foods actually cheap? Consider the long-term health consequences to you and your family. Is it worth it? The old saying "you get what you pay for" should come to mind. You will either pay for your health now—by investing in real food—or pay for disease later—by spending on doctor visits, medications, and hospital stays.

Where will you choose to spend your money?

The Price Farmers Pay for Real Food

In the United States, farmers committed to growing real food—as nature and God intended—face major expenses. Unlike food manufacturers who genetically modify crops for mass production, organic farmers grow food without modification.

Let's clear up some common misconceptions about the word *organic*:

- Organic doesn't mean farmers are doing anything extra to food to make it luxurious.
- Organic simply means the food is real—grown without genetic modification, synthetic pesticides, or artificial additives.
- Organic is different from gourmet.

Sadly, the burden of proof is on the farmers.

To label their food as organic, they must meet costly governmental requirements. And guess what? That cost gets passed onto the consumer—not because organic farmers want to overcharge you but only because the US government requires it. They must jump through dozens of hoops to prove to the US government and consumers that they simply grew their food as God intended. These hoops are quite costly, and ultimately the consumer pays *more* because our US government requires it.

The Bottom Line: Your Health Is No Place to Pinch Pennies

Consider these facts:

- Preventable illness makes up 80 percent of the burden of illness and 90 percent of all healthcare costs.
- Preventable illnesses account for eight of the nine leading categories of death.
- The United States spends more on healthcare than any other industrialized nation, yet, in many respects, its citizens are not the healthiest.[3]

These are just a few ways in which wellness is not too expensive but disease is.

I hope this will start your wheels turning—maybe even get you a little angry: you've been duped into thinking you were making the right choices, yet you keep hitting a brick wall when it comes to your health.

But now you know the truth.

In the next section, we will go even deeper—shifting your mindset and uncovering true wellness.

3 Iglehart, J.K. "The American health care system--expenditures." The New England Journal of Medicine, 340(1): January 7, 1999.

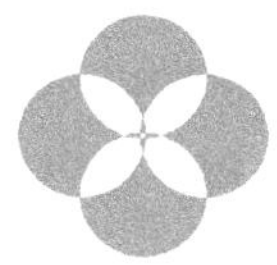

CHAPTER 3

The Paradigm Shift Continued: What Wellness Is

"Listen to advice and accept instruction, that you may gain wisdom in the future."

—Proverbs 19:20 ESV

One day, I had lunch with a director of human resources. He gave me some advice "as a friend," suggesting I needed a simpler message if I wanted to reach corporations—one that didn't come across as so anti medical.

He was right.

He used a simple analogy: Two salesmen are trying to sell him something. One has the better product, but he constantly puts down his competition, and that negativity is a turnoff.

I had to agree with him 100 percent—I don't like that approach either. I learned my lesson, hopefully at not too much of an expense.

This made me rethink my message.

My goal is not to wipe out the entire medical profession. Medicine has a purpose; it simply has little to do with true health.

I am here to share my greatest passion: the truth about wellness.

As my friend pointed out, practitioners of allopathic (i.e., traditional) medicine believe they are telling the truth about health as well.

So, how do I approach this?

I came back to something that natural health practitioners have taken issue with for years: the word *alternative*.

We have long believed that we shouldn't be the alternative—we should be the primary option.

I still believe this.

But instead of being offended by the world *alternative*, I decided to capitalize on it. After all, natural medicine, functional medicine, and wholistic healthcare truly do offer an alternative to the traditional medical model.

The difference between the two, lies only in the objective and intention of each approach.

The Difference Between Traditional Medicine and Natural Medicine

The objective of traditional medicine is to treat the disease or ailment. The method is to diagnose the condition and prescribe medications or procedures. The philosophy is linear thinking. They do this very well, and many people prefer this approach.

But natural medicine has a different objective: to get to the root cause of the problem. The method is to restore the body's natural function and bring it back to optimal health. The philosophy is to treat the whole person—mental, emotional, physical, and spiritual—simultaneously and comprehensively.

In truth, practitioners of traditional medicine are not wrong when treating the disease, but I don't believe they truly understand how to treat a person from a natural perspective. They view wellness as detecting the disease earlier and starting medication sooner, but this is not wellness; it is disease management, which is clear in the objective and semantics.

In summary, there are two models: traditional medicine and wholistic medicine. Each is an alternative to the other. Which will you choose?

Let's continue shifting your mindset about true health and wellness by examining what wellness really is.

Wellness Is a Life Change

Many years ago, my dad ended up in the hospital with diverticulitis. He had a perforation in his colon, which led to sepsis. After removing part of his intestines and keeping him in the hospital for a few days, they sent him home.

I asked, "Did they give you any dietary recommendations?"

He replied, "No, they said just don't eat strawberries."

Really?!

Either that was the only thing my dad wanted to hear or the doctors couldn't come up with any better advice than to tell him to avoid sweet, delicious, God-made strawberries.

Sadly, I have a feeling it was both. My dad didn't have the best diet or lifestyle. Maybe some people think having dinner at the bar with a couple of whiskey-and-waters beforehand—four to five nights a week—is a healthy lifestyle. Apparently, though, strawberries were the real culprit behind his diverticulitis!

There's a saying: "If you keep on doing what you've always done, you'll always get what you've always gotten!" That is the definition of insanity. You can't keep making the same choices that created your health problems and expect to get different results. Health just doesn't work that way.

If you truly want to restore your body back to good health, the first thing you need to do is to take an honest assessment of your entire health picture: mental, emotional, physical, and spiritual.

Set aside some time to write down some goals. List what needs to change in each of the four categories I mentioned above. Some areas of your health might be in better balance than others. That's okay; just start by writing *each of them* down.

- Create a heading for each quadrant of your health.
- Write at least one goal under each.
- Start small—this isn't about perfection but progress.

For example:

- **Spiritual Health**—Maybe your spiritual health is strong. Write a small goal—perhaps to deepen your relationship with God through Bible study or prayer.

- **Mental Health**—Are you overwhelmed with time management or struggling with finances, career, or purpose? Write one practical step you can take.
- **Emotional Health**—Relationships matter. What can you do to build health connections with family, friends, and coworkers?
- **Physical Health—**Assess your sleep, water intake, exercise, diet, and spinal health. Maybe instead of quitting the pub altogether, you order a healthier meal, take half home, or switch to one drink instead of several.

These goals don't have to be overwhelming or drastic. Start with small steps that can be lifelong habits.

The Power of Writing Down Goals

Financial expert Dave Ramsey teaches that his *Seven Baby Steps to Financial Freedom* are not about math—they are about psychology and emotion. The same applies to health.

Writing down goals is a huge accomplishment. It is psychologically rewarding. Studies show that written goals are significantly more likely to be achieved. We'll discuss goal setting in greater detail later. For now, just remember this: This is your moment to course-correct your health—to put your plane back on the right coordinates.

It all starts with a life change.

Wellness Is a Lifetime Commitment

Have you ever made a commitment you never intended to last a lifetime? I hear stories all the time from couples about how they first met. One person may have been more interested than the other, or perhaps one of them initially thought, "I can't stand this person—they're obnoxious. Get me away from them!" Yet, years later, they find themselves madly in love and married. They made a commitment they never expected to make—at least not at first.

There is a big difference between simply wanting something and committing to it. I could desire to be a size six, but, unless I make a real commitment (and, in my case, maybe some major plastic surgery), it's not happening!

I've known people who were living hard lives (e.g., dysfunctional relationships, addictions, homelessness); when they finally hit rock bottom, they couldn't even stand themselves any longer. Then, they rose up to *life*!

They had wanted a different life for years, but that change wouldn't happen until they made a true commitment. You need a burning commitment in your soul to do something different if you want a different result in your health—and in your life. Maybe that means making a slight improvement in one area. Maybe it means a major transformation.

Finding Your *Why*

Here are some serious questions:

Why do you want to give up junk food?

Why do you want to get more sleep?

Why do you want to end that toxic relationship once and for all?

You Need to Have a Burning Conviction in Your Spirit

Your why is what will push you to set goals, write out action steps, and follow through for a lifetime. Think long term. Think of lifelong commitment. Knowing your *why* is what turns desire into commitment.

Don't Get Swept up in the Current

Life is about making choices, sometimes on an hourly basis. It is most important to remember you have choices. That is my goal—to help you see that you have choices when it comes to your health. If you don't realize that, you could be swept up in the current of disaster. That almost happened to me.

A couple years ago, I had an appointment with a dermatologist to remove some moles. This was only the third time in twenty years that I had seen a medical doctor.

(One of those times was because I broke my leg backpacking.) I felt like a fish out of water in a doctor's office. When they asked which pharmacy I used, I told them I didn't have one. I also hadn't taken a single medication in twenty years—not even for my broken leg. It wasn't because I was trying to be difficult—I just didn't want to put something that toxic into my body. It was a choice I made.

The next day, I got a call from the nurse with the pathology report.

"You have squamous cell carcinoma," she said.

Did you cringe like I did? I *panicked.*

In an instant, I found myself falling into "patient mode."

I am not a cancer expert nor is dermatology my area of expertise. My brain started racing back to my post-doctorate days, digging through the deep, dark recesses of my memory to recall which type of skin cancer was the worst. I was walking out the door to a Christmas party when I got the news. For a moment, I got swept up into a panic and was transferred to the scheduling department to have an even bigger hole cut into my side.

Choosing to Pause, Research, and Take Control

But after I returned home several hours later, I made myself calm down, slow down, take some deep breaths, and just pause for a moment to *think* rationally and logically and draw on my own common sense and knowledge. I turned to trusted, well-respected natural health care doctors—including some MDs—and did my own research. I felt so much more at peace.

I consulted with trusted colleagues and friends who confirmed my research. I decided not to have surgery. Because cutting off a body part is like putting a piece of duct tape over the oil light in your car and thinking you fixed the problem. *You didn't*! The method does not get to the root cause.

You Always Have a Choice

Here are three major lessons I took from this experience:

1. The choice the "expert" gave me wasn't my only choice.
2. Making a rushed, fear-based decision—especially about my health—was not ideal.
3. A fear-based decision is usually the wrong decision.

A colleague once shared a powerful lesson with me: *Wait thirty days before making major decisions—about health or anything else.*

Be careful not to be swept up in the "disease current." If you lack knowledge, act out of fear, or assume you don't have a choice, you will be led down the wrong path.

You *always* have a choice.

Wellness Is Bringing the Body Back to Good Health

At the beginning of the book, we discussed the two main objectives to true wholistic health:

1. Determine the root cause
2. Restore the body back to good health

Now, let's dive deeper into that second objective.

First, you need to decide your objective. Do you want the conventional/medical approach or do you want the wholistic/natural approach? The conventional medical approach is the opposite of the wholistic natural approach.

A word of caution: It's very difficult to pursue both at the same time because they function with different objectives. Unless you are fully aware, understand how both function, and are intentional about how to integrate them, you risk conflicting treatments that may combat—rather than complement—each other.

Where to Begin?

If you feel your health isn't optimal, but you haven't reached full-blown disease, you may start by doctoring yourself.

Here's how:

- Assess your mental, emotional, physical, and spiritual health
- Rate each area on a scale from one to ten
- Set small, achievable goals for each area

Which quadrant of your health is most out of balance?

If it's physical health, evaluate these five foundational areas:

1. Rest

2. Water
3. Exercise
4. Good nutrition (minus the food-like substances)
5. Good nerve supply

Adjust accordingly, and remember—the long-range goal is to restore your body back to good health.

Track Your Progress

Use the spectrum of health to subjectively assess *your* starting point. In three months, reassess:

- Have you moved toward optimal health (i.e., left side of the spectrum)?
- Have you stayed the same?
- Have you moved toward disease (i.e., right side of the spectrum)?

If you have stayed the same or declined despite doing everything you know to do, it may be time to seek out a natural healthcare practitioner. Later in the book, we'll explore the types of practitioners available to help guide you.

But for now, be encouraged: You have made the choice to improve your health, and you *can* restore your body back to good health!

Do You Want to *Manage* Your Disease or *Restore* Your Body Back to Good Health?

Many different root causes can produce the same symptoms. Yet, mainstream medicine often fails to consider this. Instead, the message from pharmaceutical companies is "Here is your symptom, which means you have a disease, so here is your drug."

This drug is meant to be taken forever.

If a label is placed on a symptom or a group of symptoms (i.e., a complex or syndrome), there can be a drug to "cure" it—at least that's how the US government allows such drugs to be marketed.

But ask yourself:

- When was the last time you took a drug for a chronic disease and were cured (i.e., you no longer needed the drug)?
- When was the last time you heard of anyone who stopped taking medication because they were healed?

It hardly ever happens.

Most Diseases Can Be Reversed Naturally

Do you know that 75 to 80 percent of chronic degenerative diseases can be reversed naturally—without drugs? This includes:

- Diabetes
- Hypertension
- High cholesterol (which, by the way, isn't even a disease)
- Obesity
- Gallbladder problems
- Bulging discs
- Polycystic ovarian syndrome (PCOS)
- Restless leg syndrome (what is this anyway?)
- Auto-immune diseases (e.g., rheumatoid arthritis, multiple sclerosis, lupus)

- Depression
- Anxiety
- ADHD

...and the list goes on and on.

How Do You Reverse It?

First, stop looking for labels (i.e., a "disease" diagnosis).

Second, recognize symptoms are your body's way of saying something is off balance.

Remember, if you keep on doing what you've always done, you'll always get what you've always gotten.

Third, stop suppressing symptoms with drugs.

Change your behavior, and get to the root cause of the problem.

Recover your good health by:

- Changing your diet
- Exercising
- Removing nerve interference (your chiropractor can help)
- Getting more water and rest
- Addressing the spiritual and emotional aspects

This is the natural path to restoring your health. Your health *is* in your control!

Wellness Is Discipline

No one else is going to discipline you when it comes to your health. It's up to you alone. I once worked for a recovery ministry for women that focused on wholistic healing from addiction. I had the privilege of teaching wholistic health to these women. By the end of our six-week class, I saw the lightbulbs turn on in their eyes. They finally had hope—and a game plan for better health.

They made great strides toward healing their bodies naturally, making healthy food choices, exercising, letting go of the diet sodas, and so much more. It was exciting to see the physical changes and mental determination in them. Their skin was clearer, their eyes were brighter, they had more energy, they started dropping a few pounds, and they had greater mental clarity.

Then *boom*—reality hit.

A graduation, holiday, or special event rolled around. People brought sweets and junk food; just like that, their discipline was challenged. Sugary processed foods trigger the same addiction pathways in the brain as drugs and alcohol.

For someone in recovery, this can be a dangerous setback. If you know someone walking out of addiction recovery, please:

- Do not bring them sweets or processed foods
- Instead, support their discipline with healthier options

I once heard a political candidate explain how he stayed true to his morals. He said, "When I am getting ready to take a lady out on a date, if I don't have it in my mind ahead of time how I will treat her with the utmost respect and integrity, then I will be setting myself up to tremendous weakness and caving into my unwise desires and choices."

That stuck with me. It applies not only to moral decisions but also to dietary choices.

If you don't decide your food convictions ahead of time, you will cave.

Know your absolutes:

- No gluten
- No sugar
- No empty carbs
- No sodas

Be mentally prepared to say no—to yourself *and* others. Wellness takes discipline; plan for it.

I was brought up by a mom who was raised by a Depression-era mother. The "don't throw food away" mentality and a mindset of lack was passed down from generation to generation. I also went to Catholic grade school in the 1960s and 1970s. The nuns would stand by the garbage cans in the cafeteria to make sure students wouldn't throw anything other than apple cores and paper products into the waste can. There were poor kids around the world starving to death, you know! Now, while this is most certainly true, that is no justification to feel obligated to eat for *every* starving child. I have lived most of my life eating everything on my plate, including the huge portions served to me at every restaurant I've visited. It takes much discipline to change this mentality and let go of the guilt I was encouraged to carry at the risk of my own health.

Another good strategy to avoid caving into poor food choices is to carry alternate foods with you. I attend many breakfast meetings and networking events. I overcome caving to the temptation of breakfast sandwiches and pastries by eating breakfast at home before I leave the house. Wellness takes discipline, so plan for it.

Wellness Is Your Insurance

So far, we've learned our health is our responsibility alone—not our insurance company's, not our employer's, and certainly not our government's. We also covered that *health insurance* is a misnomer; if we don't recognize this and start to call it what it really is (i.e., medical insurance), we might find ourselves far off course from our objective. Assuming your objective is to restore your body back to good health, or even to maintain your health, you must begin viewing your insurance for the purpose of "in case something happens" to your health and understand you actually desire medical insurance rather than health insurance.

To solidify this perspective, let's explore ways of using our medical insurance the same way we use our car insurance. When shopping for car insurance, we are typically given the option of a $500 or $1,000 deductible, which includes what we are responsible for and the initial cost for repairs as well as similar costs. Our choice is likely based on several considerations. First, we consider our savings and salary. Keep in mind the policy with a $1,000 deductible will require a lower monthly premium (i.e., the amount paid for the benefit of having insurance) than the policy with a $500 deductible. Second, we consider how often we might put our policy to use by assessing factors such as past car accidents, the amount of time we spend driving, our level of experience behind the wheel, and the reliability of our reflexes. Finally, we choose a policy based on these considerations. Ideally, we will never use this insurance, but it's available should we need it.

Car insurance doesn't cover regular car maintenance like oil changes, tire replacement, brake replacement, and many other things we *should* do if we want to maintain the longevity of the car. It also doesn't cover unexpected repairs like a blown gasket, bad wheel bearings, burning oil, a leak in the radiator, and a tire puncture. All these things can be minimized, if not avoided, if we take care of the car through routine maintenance and repair.

Now, let's apply this concept to our health or medical insurance. The general state of your health, as well as the steps you take to maintain it, can help you choose the right deductible for your medical insurance. Your choices may be limited if you receive your medical insurance through your employer, but you can still benefit from this knowledge and make decisions about your health accordingly. In fact, truly considering and respecting your employer and your coworkers means keeping costs down by taking responsibility for your health. In a group plan, everyone pays for everyone else's lack of responsibility.

Take responsibility for your health—take ownership of it—as if it were a car. Maintain your body and health with rest, water, exercise, good nutrition, and good nerve supply. These foundations of health are analogous to the routine maintenance performed on cars. In fact, my car (like most cars) has an owner's manual that tells me how often to service each component. It even includes a log to record the date of each service. You can do the same for your body! I suggest performing a quick monthly assessment for each area of your health and setting quarterly goals set in each area of your physical foundation.

If something doesn't seem quite right with your body, have it checked out—just like you should do with your car. If the oil light lit up on the dashboard of your car, would you have it checked out, or would you put a piece of black tape over it and trust that the problem had been solved because you can't see the light any longer?

Of course you would have it checked out! In fact, most of us would do so immediately. We might not (and should not) drive one more mile with that light on. How much more important and valuable is your body?

This is where medical and car insurance differ and my analogy begins to fail. Medical insurance rarely covers checkups. If your insurance covers checkups, take advantage of your coverage before matters get worse. A visit to a medical doctor or specialist can help nip something in the bud and is far less costly than winding up in the hospital. For most people, however, such visits are very costly, even including insurance.

When I had a CT scan in 2022 for what turned out to be a kidney stone, the imaging revealed a benign ovarian teratoma cyst. I had no symptoms. If not for that CT scan, I might have gone the rest of my life unaware of it. On the other hand, I might have been in big trouble if the cyst had ruptured or started torquing around another body part internally.

I backpack regularly in the wilderness, sometimes alone. I certainly would not have wanted that kind of trouble while in the wilderness. I made the wise decision to have it removed before matters got worse. I was thankful for having medical insurance. This was a true medical need, and there was nothing I could have done to prevent this. The cyst had probably been there since birth, and it wasn't due to me not taking care of my health.

At my post-surgery visit, the gynecologist showed me some pictures taken internally during the laparoscopic surgery. I was thankful to hear that everything looked great internally—nice and pink and healthy! But would her report have been the same if I were not so conscious of maintaining my health? Possibly not. Fortunately, this was not an emergency surgery, and I had time to think and pray about the direction I wanted to take. My wellness complemented my medical insurance, so I could receive this positive report.

Wellness Is Common-Sense Simple

Hopefully, by now, you are starting to understand that our health and how we take care of it—even restore it—is simple common-sense. When we got in the plane and set our coordinates, we were deceived into setting them a degree or two off course; now, many years later, we find ourselves misguided and off course to common sense. That is the purpose of this book: to shed light on the truth that has been robbed from most of us.

The solution is to get back on track by following the most common-sense, least expensive, and simplest protocols to take care of our health. I am not a statistician, but I have researched and learned a great deal about these simple protocols. In my heart and mind, I know that following them faithfully can lower the cost of healthcare and prevent most chronic diseases. The sooner in life we start, the better off we will be.

To recap, these basic protocols consist of *regular* exercise; drinking good, clean water; eating chemical-free fruits and vegetables and other real foods; getting seven to nine hours of uninterrupted sleep each night; and making sure your body has good nerve supply.

We need to become conscious of the dependent, fast-paced mentality that tells us our health is someone else's responsibility so these basic protocols don't seem so foreign to us. Good health occurs only by addressing each of these protocols. No one else can do these things for you. Take some time to understand the big picture of where you and our society have been headed throughout the past fifty years or more—away from simple common sense. How has that been working for us? I encourage you to take a deep breath, slow down, and simply start by taking one step at a time, one day at a time, in the right direction.

Wellness Is Freedom

Once you adopt this paradigm shift in your thinking, you can start putting the plane back on its correct course—this should be freeing to you! Hopefully the lightbulb of hope is at least becoming a glimmer in your eye. My prayer is that you are breathing easier, becoming energized, and feeling a stir of hope in your spirit!

It is helpful to think wholistically—not linearly—about your health. Linear thinking is typical of traditional medicine: when a patient has a pain/symptom in a body part, the doctor looks at that part and gives the "magic" prescription/pill or—even worse—removes the body part. This is "outward, inward" thinking, which does not identify the root cause of the problem.

Remember, wholistic health comes from God (above) and from within; the integrity of our bodies' internal environment determines our health. Always ask yourself what the root cause of the problem is rather than looking to address the symptom. The symptom is just your body's way of telling you something is out of balance. You need to commit to a continual discovery mission to determine the source of your body's imbalance and steps you can take to correct it. Think wholistically—mental (e.g., time management, budget, goal setting, career, purpose), emotional, physical, and spiritual. The root cause can lie in any of those arenas.

As you begin thinking wholistically to identify the root cause of your problem and make positive changes, you will notice quick improvements in many aspects of your health, including blood sugar, energy levels, quality of sleep, libido, mood, blood pressure, internal body temperature, clarity of thinking, and so much more! Even joint pain and body aches can diminish. When you commit to wholistic thinking, you will find yourself on the course toward disease prevention and optimum health.

Once again, *your health is in your control*! Be empowered with this knowledge and these truths. Believe this and start walking it out.

Call to Action: Chapters 2 and 3 thoroughly examine the ways in which we use and think about certain words. Perhaps you have doubted your words can really influence your health, but they do have an effect. It's a big-picture view of what has been indoctrinated in us for years. A paradigm shift in your thinking is an excellent place to start making changes. I encourage you to pay attention to what you hear, read, and see when it comes to health. Ask yourself "Is this truly health? Or is this just managing disease?" Make a note of your observations or share them with a friend.

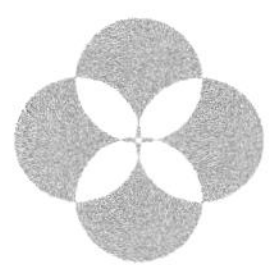

CHAPTER 4

Caring for Your Spiritual, Mental, and Emotional Health

"I am but a pilgrim here on earth: how I need a map–and your commands are my chart and guide. I long for your instructions more than I can tell."

—Psalm 119:19-20 TLB

On March 6, 1996, when God delivered me from an addiction to alcohol, smoking, the whole bar lifestyle, I had been reading some self-help books, one of which was *What to Say When You Talk to Yourself* by Dr. Shad Helmstetter. I have no idea how I came across this book—internet search engines were in their infancy, and Amazon certainly wasn't on my radar. Nevertheless, it was a truly pivotal seed that started me on my wholistic transformational journey.

Although I didn't know it at the time, God was prompting me to start my wholistic journey of changing my spiritual, mental, emotional, and physical health. Deciding to change my career, I took a career assessment course (mental health). I wanted to help others along this amazing journey and wondered what kind of career would help me do so. I sought family counseling for myself (emotional health). I focused on my physical health and started going to the gym and changing my horrible eating habits (think convenience store burritos, topped with extra cheese, at 4:00 a.m., *before* going to bed!). Not by coincidence, I attended a women's church retreat (spiritual health) with a woman from my women's pool league. She and I had played pool together at a local bar. See how God can truly use His people anywhere? At the time, I thought this was my own, newly created philosophy of wholistic health, but I later learned this approach to health went much further back than 1996!

Using the wisdom that God has given each of us to help maintain and restore our health has been acknowledged and implemented for centuries. In fact, as far back as 400 BC, Hippocrates, the "father of medicine," said to his students, "Let thy food be thy medicine and thy medicine be thy food." He also said, "A wise man should consider that health is the greatest of human blessings." These two statements could be neither truer nor more relevant to the message of this book.

The World Health Organization (WHO) defines health as "a state of complete physical, mental, and social well-being and not merely the absence of disease or infirmity." More accurately, optimum wellness requires mental, emotional, physical, and spiritual health to be balanced and functioning optimally. When one of these areas is out of balance, that imbalance affects the others, as they are all interconnected and related. Focusing on one area while ignoring the others will eventually lead to a state of "dis-ease," imbalance, and ultimately sickness. For example, if a person is always angry (emotional health), they just might end up having a heart attack (physical health). If someone has unforgiveness in their heart (spiritual health), they will more than likely find it quite difficult to achieve optimum physical health. If someone is trying to fit twenty-eight hours into a twenty-four-hour day (mental health), their physical health will suffer as well.

Before moving on, let's review some key concepts. It's important to understand the differences between traditional medicine's approach to health and wellness and the wholistic/natural approach. Envision the spectrum of health we discussed in chapter 2.

On the left side of the line is 100 percent health, and on the right side is 99 percent disease (100 percent disease indicates death). When a doctor tells a patient their lab work numbers are "fine," that person generally assumes they are on the far-left side of this spectrum of health (i.e., 100 percent healthy). That's amazing, but health isn't merely the absence of disease. This method of viewing health overlooks the large gap between the left and right sides of the spectrum; most of us fall within this large middle area! Traditional medicine is linear—you are either diseased or healthy, with no place between. The wholistic approach looks at a person's health as a whole, considering all factors and avoiding black/white, yes/no, and either/or approaches. Our objective is to get to the root cause of the problem and work toward restoring the body to good health using natural and wholistic approaches.

Health Is Not Linear

To benefit from the spectrum of health, first gather *all* possible data. Avoid labeling yourself as diseased or not diseased based on one or two numbers. For starters, determine your current position along the spectrum of health (i.e., your starting point) then aim toward the left end of the spectrum (i.e., optimum health).

Second, consider your whole health: mental, emotional, physical, and spiritual. This is a big-picture view of health, which I call the *whole health pie*. Within the physical quadrant of the health pie, five pieces are significantly foundational and vital to optimal health. These are rest, water, exercise, good nutrition/minus the toxins (i.e., consuming valuable nutrients rather than harmful, toxic substances), and good nerve supply.

The following sections define the four basic quadrants of the wholistic health pie.

Quadrant 1: Spiritual Health

While all the pieces of the health pie are vital, most factors hinge on our spiritual health. It's the measuring stick, the origin of truth for all other aspects of our health. It manifests our relationship with the One Who created us and breathed the breath of life into us.

Don't get me wrong: our spiritual health cannot stay balanced if we ignore the other parts of our health—they are all vital. God created us in His *whole* image—mental, emotional, physical, and spiritual. Ignoring the other parts means ignoring part of Him. This results in a spiritual health imbalance. It is therefore essential to start with spiritual health.

A vital tool for our entire health is your ability to hear God's voice and your confidence in that ability. His voice will direct us toward keeping (or bringing) all the areas of our health into balance. I've gleaned many of my insights about spiritual health from a wholistic approach from Drs. Mark and Patti Virkler's *4 Keys to Hearing God's Voice* (Destiny Image Publishers, 2010), an excellent resource for learning to hear God's voice. God communicates His plans for you by speaking directly to you—hearing Him is vital to your health and direction in life.

Dr. Virkler expertly describes the four simple steps to hearing God's voice:

1. Quiet yourself down
2. Picture yourself with Jesus (or Papa God)
3. Be open to spontaneous thoughts and visions
4. Write it down—journal what you hear or see

Once I committed to these four basic steps, my relationship with Jesus deepened immensely! There is nothing sweeter than starting your day by seeking direction from the One who has already mapped out your steps—not for the day but rather your entire earthly existence! He is waiting for you to turn to Him and intimately converse with Him every day!

For a greater understanding of Drs. Virkler's *How to Hear God's Voice*, See Appendix B at the end of the book.

A Word from the Lord

I believe with all my heart that God has called me to speak, write, and teach on wholistic health and wellness. I have journaled some of the things the Lord has spoken to me throughout the years, and I've applied the principles of hearing God's voice to my own life, specifically concerning my passion for teaching others the truth about health and wellness. Here is one of those journal entries:

> *Lord, will you tell me and show me what You want me to say to the Church regarding their health?*

> *Keep it simple. You have such a passion for their health that you want to tell them everything, leaving no stone unturned. This can be overwhelming for them—at least in a sermon opportunity. Begin by laying out the foundation of mental, emotional, physical, and spiritual health. Tell them that it is important to get to the root. Tell them it is important to be able to hear My Voice. I want you to take this message first to the spirit-filled Church. Remind them that they are free, and that I sent My Son Jesus to FULFILL the Law—tell them what that means, using the teaching I gave you about this. Be sure they know you are not coming from a place of legalism but from a place of responsibility. Tell them how oppressed the Church is and that I want them FREE! Then tell them the vision I showed you and what I told you when you asked Me what I saw. Tell them and show them that the Church without the Spirit is dead, but the same is true when the Church doesn't take responsibility for its physical health. Emphasize the importance to them about bringing their bodies back to good health naturally. Share with them James 2—study this now and meditate on it so you will know what I mean and what I want you to share with them. They must be convinced that it is My desire for them to take care of their health before they will do it. I want you to convince them of this.*

One evening, I discovered a Christian believer's website. Its creator seemed very passionate about natural health and quoted Bible passages regarding the care of our temples. His words were true, but as I continued to explore his website, I realized a crucial component was missing—supernatural healing! The Holy Spirit seemed to be absent from his beliefs regarding the health of the Christian. The next morning, the Lord spoke the following to my heart:

Good morning, Lord. Lord, as I was lying in bed, you were showing me where some division lies within the Church in regard to our whole health. Some believe that it is vitally important to take care of our (physical) health as You have laid out in the Bible, but they don't acknowledge supernatural healings (spiritual). This is one end of the spectrum, typically the mainstream denominational churches, (e.g., Presbyterians, Lutherans, Baptists, Seventh Day Adventists). Then there are those on the other end of the spectrum who believe in nothing but supernatural healings; they take no responsibility for their physical health (e.g., Pentecostals, Charismatics). This is why I am not seeing enough comprehensive teachings on health, nor am I seeing people healthy and whole! There are also a whole lot of mixed signals in each of these camps. The Charismatics believe in healings, but in the meantime, they don't give a second thought to taking drugs until You heal them! They won't take responsibility for themselves (slothfulness). The religious believers like rules, discipline, and doctrine so they will emphasize strict practices in diet and exercise (works), and they will pray for God to heal them, but they don't believe healing is ALREADY theirs; they think it's a "maybe, maybe not" chance. Wow, this is becoming so clear to me—keep speaking to me, Lord, keep speaking to me! This is "works" vs. the "spiritualists." Dr. Virkler made a similar comparison when he talked about Phariseeism versus New Age. Wow, thank You, Lord, for showing me this division. Now I need You to show me the teaching to convict both—or at least the spiritualists—on the truth about health. I am thinking of the whole health approach as marketplace health and healing. Show me in Your Word, Lord, where both are

> *vital for optimal health and healing. This is the foundation for the approach I need to take the teachings to the Church. The spiritualists think natural health is New Age and the work folks think the Holy Spirit is not for today—so we are throwing stones at each other from each direction! Show me how to break through to them, Lord!*
>
> *"You are dealing with unbelief from both sides. You are also dealing with rebellion, slothfulness, and of course a spirit of religion. Faith without works is dead. Study this teaching* (James 2:14-17 NASB) *in its proper context."*

I studied these scriptures and I found the following:

> "What use is it, my brethren, if someone says he has faith but he has no works? Can that faith save him?" James 2:14.

In this case, *works* means an act, deed, effort, or doing. The word *save* means to deliver or protect, heal, preserve, save (self), do well, and be (make) whole.

What good is the healing line or your faith that the Holy Spirit will heal you if you take no individual action to support that healing? Will this faith heal, protect, preserve, or make you whole again?

For example, if you were to witness someone delivered from a spirit of addiction to alcohol (faith), you would certainly advise them to avoid places that may tempt them to return to their addiction.

> "If a brother or sister is without clothing and in need of daily food, and one of you says to them 'go in peace, be warmed and be filled,' and yet you do not give them

> what is necessary for their body, what use is that?" James 2:15–16

If we treat others this way, we should treat ourselves the same. If a healing minister prays for you to heal, and you believe you are healed, what good is that belief if you do not maintain your healing with good nourishment, water, exercise, and words of life?

> "Even so faith, if it has no works, is dead, being by itself." James 2:17

We need to back up our faith with action! What is this *action*?

For starters, we must assess our health as a whole—mental, emotional, physical, and spiritual. Determine which quadrant of your health pie identifies the root cause of your problem, address it appropriately, and return the body to good health and balance using natural approaches. All areas of our health are interrelated—if one is out of balance, others will be also.

This is not about legalism. You are not a sinner if you don't take care of your health, and you won't get a free ticket to Heaven if you do! Father God simply wants you and me to be free from sickness and disease while on this earth. If you do get sick, you should not feel guilty or condemned—after all, we live in a fallen, imperfect world; let no one tell you you're not good enough or that you did something wrong. Spiritual health has nothing to do with shame. It's simply about stewarding the only body God has given us, and He has provided the tools to show and tell us how to do so.

After studying James as God instructed me to, He then spoke these words to me:

> *"I see a dependence on things other than Me, like drugs and medications. I see fear, I see gluttony, I see manipulation and control and deception by the food and drug companies. I see irresponsibility in not taking care of the body, My Temple I gave and created for each child of Mine. I see abuse of these bodies. This abuse is caused both by the person themselves as well as inflicted by others—this too causes a lack of caring for their Temples. I see a lack of trust in Me to take care of them—not after the fact but instead of. For example, they will eat foods made by man because they are fast, easy, and cheap, rather than eating foods I made for them like fruits, vegetables, grains, and yes, even meats and eggs. They do not slow down long enough to minister to their Temples; they don't slow down to spend time with Me. They are depending on so many other things rather than Me. Food is their god. Poor time management is a real problem. I also see slothfulness and laziness. All these things hurt My heart and are not My plans for them. They are so ingrained in the so-called comforts of the world that they no longer enjoy the pleasures I made for them. I made my beauty all around them, all things of the earth and sky, land and water, good food from these places, and so much more. Simpleness has been lost—everything is go, go, go."*

The core tenet of the Christian faith is the Holy Trinity: God the Father, God the Son (i.e., Jesus Christ), and God the Holy Spirit. Father God sent His Son, Jesus Christ, to walk this earth as a human so we might hear, see, and learn the truth about Heavenly Father's love for us with our own eyes and ears through Jesus. In essence, Father God, the God of the Bible, brought Himself to earth in human form to demonstrate His love for us; through Jesus Christ, we can reunite with the Father for eternity. He did this by allowing Jesus to be crucified on the cross—the most horrendous death anyone could possibly imagine—to take not only our sins to His grave but also our sickness and disease once and for all; "by His stripes we *are* healed." (Isaiah 53:5 NKJV).

The Holy Spirit guides and empowers us daily throughout our lives. The Father wants us to walk in freedom! We are set free from all that binds us—mentally, emotionally, physically, and spiritually—not only because He loves us but also because Jesus died for us. Whether you are a believer in the Christian faith or not, I encourage you to study these truths—and all the truths this book contains—for your own peace of mind. Truth begins when the Christian believer models all the truths of the Lord, including that of health. Only then can truth be carried to all people.

The Truth about the Words We Speak

To paraphrase Proverbs 23:7, as a man thinks in his heart so he becomes. This is how we own our disease. Stop saying *my* diabetes, *my* gout, *my* celiac, *my* cancer. I have met far too many people whose identities lie within their diagnosed diseases, and it truly breaks my heart. Most chronic degenerative diseases can be *reversed.* When they say they have diabetes, for example, they speak with an air of ownership—like their disease is a badge of honor or battle scar. It's almost as if they are saying, with their chests puffed out, "Yep, it's my diabetes. It's mine now, and nobody better try to take it away from me—I've been tagged as another victim." When I tell them they need not live with disease for the rest of their lives, they look a little deflated. In many cases, they look shocked; too often, they quickly choose not to believe me. I speak the truth over you: your health is in *your* control! As a man thinks in his heart so he becomes.

The words we speak to others influence our health. If someone is trying to restore their body to good health by avoiding foods that are not good for the body, don't try talking them into eating that piece of cake! This is like trying to convince an alcoholic with six years of sobriety to take a drink! Respect their journey to good health.

I took a seminar several years ago, and the instructor would get annoyed with questions regarding specific diseases. He said the body doesn't know it's diagnosed with diabetes, for example; it only knows it is out of balance and not functioning optimally. Drug companies classify symptoms as diseases so they can develop a drug to treat them. When a patient or customer would tell me they had a particular disease, I wouldn't follow them down that rabbit hole, chasing after the so-called disease or symptom(s). Instead, I would go back to the basics and look for the root cause of the imbalance before helping them bring the body back into balance.

I encourage you to do the same; don't own the diagnosis your doctor assigns you. Instead, press the medical practitioner a little when they give you a diagnosis. Ask them which factors led to that conclusion. Ask for a root cause. Don't settle for an unknown cause—baloney! Ask how their recommendations address the root cause. Ask whether their suggested protocol intends to restore the body to balance and good health or simply change the symptoms or lab values. Hear the diagnosis then take control of your health and your life and work toward bringing the body back into balance using natural approaches. Invite them to walk alongside you toward this objective. If they are unable to do so, seek out a practitioner who will. Drugs prescribed for thousands of diseases will not reverse a diagnosis—they only manage it. Your disease or imbalance *can* be eliminated or reversed when you approach it wholistically.

When her patients said they were "catching a cold," a dear friend of mine would tell them, "Then put your hand down and quit catching it!" If you are diagnosed with a disease, the first thing you should do is stand up and speak the truth: "I *will not* have this for long. I am taking control of my health." If you don't plan on changing your lifestyle, you must follow your doctor's orders by all means. If you want to be rid of the diagnosed problem and are willing to make a commitment to take control of your health, engage your mental health, make a plan, and set some goals and action steps to achieve control.

In many ways, I find it hard to pray for most people when they request a healing prayer for their chronic degenerative diseases. In my mind, they are unlikely to change their ways, which most likely caused their disease. It hurts my heart to see people pray at the altar for healing from chronic disease then leave the church service for an all-you-can-eat buffet or a similar restaurant. I believe God often has answers to their prayers and heals them at the altar, but they abandon His gift the moment they continue making poor lifestyle choices.

I am not saying my attitude is right. Quite often, I must repent and ask God for a more compassionate heart, a less judgmental heart, a heart full of grace. I *do* pray that God gives them wisdom of the truth about their sickness, what has caused it, and how to change it. After all, health and healing are wholistic, and wisdom applies to the spiritual and mental areas of the health pie. Wisdom and commitment can lead to action in addressing the root cause of the problem, wherever that root may be. If we all focus our healing prayers a little more wholistically, we just might experience greater healing and health.

Whether we succeed in taking control of our health and reversing these chronic degenerative diseases has depended a great deal on our attitudes and the words we speak. The Bible does not say that we will get a disease and die. It is we who have declared this falsehood by predicting how we will die. "Diabetes runs in my family; my mom died of it, so I probably will too." Hogwash! Discussing faith, the Bible also says, ". . . call those things which do not exist as though they did" (Romans 4:17 NKJV). Start speaking life over yourself and your family instead of sickness, disease, and death. Start picturing yourself as healthy and whole—mentally, emotionally, physically, and spiritually. Our health is a lifetime process, and it is in our control to a large degree. Take control of it! We make choices every day, so why choose to picture, think, and talk about the negative when you can just as easily choose the positive? "Death and life are in the power of the tongue . . ." (Proverbs 18:21 NKJV). Choose *life*!

Quadrant 2: Mental Health

Mental health concerns things like time management, budget, career, goal setting, and purpose in life. Do we even know why we get out of bed in the morning? If not, why should we care if we are healthy? Most people say they don't have enough time or money to take better care of their health.

This is why it is so important to address our health as a whole rather than looking at our physical health alone to fix the problem. The true root cause of diabetes, for example, can be deeper than your glucose levels being too high. Taking the time to prepare healthy meals would help lower your blood glucose.

In the next section, I give some examples of mental health and explain how each plays a part in overall wholistic health.

The Truth about Planning

Have you ever heard the adage "if you fail to plan, you plan to fail"? I have observed my own behavior from time to time, especially around the holidays or busier-than-usual times at work, and I will eat anything that is quick and easy if I don't *plan* my meals. After all, I'm hungry! Dinner seems to be the hardest for me. For others, it might be breakfast or lunch. Do you head for the nearest drive-through for a fast-food breakfast sandwich or rely on vending machines or frozen meals instead of planning your lunch? This leaves many feeling guilty, tired, bloated, and frustrated, which leads to giving up on living a healthier lifestyle once again. The vicious cycle continues.

The mental part of our wholistic health involves setting goals. When I was in chiropractic school, our schooling was scheduled quarterly, so I began setting quarterly goals. Three months is not too long or too short. You have enough time to reach your goal without allowing too many unknown variables to keep you from achieving them. (Short-term goals can be your action steps to long-term goals.) I learned about writing down things like objectives, goals, and action steps many years before as an administrative assistant for a professional association. It was a wonderful learning experience for me at twenty-five years old, and I've carried it ever since.

First, you need to write down your objective(s). Ask yourself why you want to reach your goal (i.e., your motivation). In my late forties, I gained 30 pounds while going through menopause—and I was training for a marathon at the time! I had never had a weight problem. I might have gained a few pounds here and there, but with a little dietary change and exercise, I had always been able to bring my weight back on track. I needed to understand this and get to the root cause. My motivation wasn't just personal—even more so, it was professional and based on my passion to help others with their health. If I couldn't lose weight and help myself, how could I help others? My objective was to learn the root causes of weight gain and how to lose weight so I could help others.

Next, write down your goal. I suggest writing a goal or two in each quadrant of your health—mental, emotional, physical, and spiritual. If your goal is to lose 30 pounds, for example, the key is to *write it down*. It may seem trivial, and you may think you don't have to write down your goal since you already know it. But writing it down is *key*! Make sure you can see it all the time. I write my goals in a Microsoft Word file saved to my laptop—the same file I've used for many years. Each goal *must* also have a completion date (e.g., I will reach this goal by________)."

Now, write down your action steps. These capture how you are going to reach this goal. *This* is where planning becomes so important. Your action steps need to be specific. For example, the action steps for eating a more alkalized diet begin with identifying alkalized foods (e.g., fruits, vegetables, nuts and seeds, good fats, and water) and avoiding others (e.g., fast food, fried foods, packaged processed foods, and sugar). (I'll discuss each of these foods in the physical health section.) The next step is finding new recipes. (If you need to lose 30 pounds, your old recipes obviously don't work!)

To follow these recipes, you may need to shop for ingredients at a health food store, which many people find unfamiliar. Don't underestimate this as a potential barrier to achieving your goals. Often, we don't like stepping out of our comfort zone. Have you ever shopped at an unfamiliar grocery store on vacation? You felt lost in there, didn't you? When you can't zip in and out, your shopping takes longer. Prepare yourself for setbacks as you work toward your goal; changing the way you cook or shop slows you down at first. It's okay—you will achieve a new, healthier routine soon enough!

The first time I committed to a vegetarian diet, I was in chiropractic school. All the "tree huggers" were doing it, so I decided to as well. I was going to make some scones, and the recipe called for currants. I had never heard of—let alone eaten—a scone, not to mention a currant! I had to humble myself at a local health food store by asking, "Sir, please excuse my ignorance, but *where* might I find your currants and *what* are they?" I didn't know what currants *looked like* or which aisle I should check! But the next time, I knew.

If we want to change our lives—whether mentally, physically, spiritually, or emotionally—we need a *plan* to do so, and we must write it down with an "achieve by" date. This makes the difference between simply *desiring* to do something and *committing* to do it. You can achieve what you want when you follow these action steps. Believe me, it works. I lost 25 of the 30 pounds I had gained by simply changing to a more alkalizing diet. I committed to it instead of wishing for it, and I had a plan. You too can achieve your goals. If you fall off the horse, you haven't failed; it's never too late to get back on. To paraphrase Robert Schuller, failure is not falling; failure is simply failing to get back up. So make a plan!

The Truth About Budgets

When my mother and I discussed her health, it was always the same. She would go to the doctor, and I'd ask, "What did the doctor say?" She would say, "I don't know. I don't understand him, but he said to take this prescription." I'd ask, "What's it for?" She'd reply, "I don't know, Jack" (short for Jackie). I would then replace my Jack hat with my doctor hat, suggesting some natural remedies. Her first resistance was, "Will my insurance cover it?" Of course, the answer was no, and that would be that. My response to her, you, and myself "don't let the insurance company dictate the level of your health!"

Two huge factors of our mental health that can throw the rest out of balance or into a diseased state: time and money. "I don't have enough time" and "I don't have enough money" are the two most common phrases people use to resist my health advice. I once used them as well. We must all remain conscious of the risk of resisting or making excuses. Juliet B. Schor has written two books that recognize this problem: *The Overworked American* and *The Overspent American.*

We spend our time and money on our priorities. For example, consider the ten "yeah, buts" from chapter 2; this is a matter of priorities. Some of my chiropractic patients would claim they couldn't afford the care plan I suggested. I so desperately believed in my approach and felt so sorry for them that I reduced my fees, making sure they knew their health would continue to decline without good nerve supply. Several weeks later, they would tell me about their upcoming Alaskan cruise. I thought they were broke! I'm sure if we were truly honest with ourselves, we could say we've all been there, on both the receiving end and on the delivery of that message.

Even the poorest in this country can receive some kind of financial support—particularly food stamps. The problem here lies partly with the federal government, which approves food stamps for cheap, food-like substances like sodas, snack/junk food, and other sugar-laden drinks. Recipients of these benefits can also buy organic fruits, vegetables, and other groceries if they choose. Unfortunately, food stamps go a lot further when utilized to buy sugar and food-like substances. I wonder what would happen to our society and the health of its citizens if food stamps only applied to fruits, vegetables, nuts and seeds, good fats, and water.

Those using food stamps or on a very tight budget should first have a written budget for groceries each week or month. Food should be one of the top priorities on the budget, along with housing and transportation needs. These priorities must be "needs" rather than "wants." Many people *want* to live in a mansion, drive a Maserati, and dine on lobster and caviar, but these are not needs. It's important to plan your menu for the week and know your budget. Start with a nutritionally dense menu. If that means simply eating various vegetables for breakfast, lunch, and dinner, so be it. No one has ever died of eating too many vegetables. However, many have died of eating a high-calorie, low-nutrition diet, at least when consumed over many years. This describes the typical American diet, no matter how rich or poor someone is.

The Truth about Our Purpose

Years ago, when I first turned my life around and realized there was more to life than just sitting in dark, dingy barrooms night after night, I was invited to a picnic. The atmosphere was the typical bar-crowd picnic: good food, drinks galore, and the usual talk about the latest music and the fastest boat. Unknown to them, I was mentally, emotionally, and spiritually moving in a new and different direction with my life. I was coming to the realization that I had a purpose in life, one that went way beyond sitting in barrooms every night. I struck up a conversation with one man by asking, "How long do you want to live?" His reply (sadly) was, "Oh, maybe sixty-five." Most of us were probably in our mid-thirties, some maybe a little older. But sixty-five? I recall asking him if he didn't want to live long enough to see his grandchildren grow up. The look on his face seemed to say that thought wasn't even on his radar; in fact, it almost seemed unimaginable to him. This man clearly didn't even know he had a purpose.

We all have a unique, divine reason for being on this earth. Years ago, I gave a speech on this topic at my Toastmasters Club in Charleston, South Carolina. I used the phrase "unique, *divine* reason." As is the nature of Toastmasters meetings, I had an evaluator for my speech—a young man, maybe in his mid-twenties. One of his critiques was to not use the word "divine," as it might offend some people. Again, how sad. Who does he think our purpose comes from? For whom are we fulfilling it? The answer to both questions is God. If you don't believe this, it is understandable that you don't believe you have a purpose and perhaps are offended by the use of the word "divine." But you do, and it is from Him.

Unfortunately, even those inside the Christian church don't all know they have a purpose. And for those who do, some don't know what that purpose is. I can appreciate not knowing, but I highly encourage you to continue to press into God and ask Him what it is. What is the passion that burns in your heart when someone is wronged?

Do you even know why you get out of bed in the morning? If you don't have a solid reason for more than just life's necessities, what do you care whether you are mentally, physically, emotionally, or spiritually healthy? That's why all the pieces of the health pie are connected and interrelated—each influences the others.

You have a purpose. You matter—not just to God but also to your family, friends, coworkers, and community. You are valuable, and we need you. Without you, we all fall a little short in our purpose. We need each other for a healthier community and a healthier body of Christ.

Quadrant 3: Emotional Health

Wholistic health comprises our spiritual, mental, emotional, and physical health. One area cannot stand independent from the others, whether for better or worse.

My Story

At nine years old, I began to have a lot of cramping, pain, and poor bowel movements. This went on for some time until I was finally admitted to the hospital for an overnight stay. The doctors wanted to sedate me for an internal exam the next day. It was frightening to be admitted into the hospital without either parent to stay with me through the night, especially since I did not understand why I had been admitted.

I was ultimately diagnosed with mild colitis, a digestive imbalance that causes inflammation in the large intestine and a severe diagnosis for a child. I was told to avoid milk due to a likely sensitivity.

I do not believe milk was the root cause of my illness today. I now believe several factors made me so sick, including:

1) **Diet**: I was raised during the fast food and processed food boom of the 1960s and 1970s. I ate a lot of sugar and drank a lot of milk. We now know that cow's milk is the number one hidden food sensitivity. It is very inflammatory and very mucous forming—both of which mimic a colitis diagnosis.
2) **Stress**: My daily life was filled with emotional stress. My mom and dad often raised their voices to each other and their four kids. If one of us did something wrong, we were all punished. I recall being sent to the basement (where, as a child, I had

fears of monsters getting me) on more than one occasion to stay until I stopped crying.

But this was just the beginning of my digestive challenges. At sixteen years old, I was working a part-time job after school at a five-and-dime store that sold all kinds of little trinkets as well as candy bars. I probably spent half my paycheck on candy bars to eat while I was working. I also had access to candy bars at home; my dad owned a vending machine business, and we truly had an endless supply of candy bars, which I often ate after dinner for years.

I recall having to leave work early on more than one occasion because my gut was cramping up so bad that the only way to relieve the pain was to lie flat on my stomach for 30 minutes or so. I was the only employee working, and I had to call the owner to come and relieve me. She wasn't very happy with me, causing even more stress.

My digestive problems continued into my twenties and thirties as I entered the dysfunctional world of drinking and bar life, living a life of unhealthy relationships without a purpose or direction. At the time, I didn't make any connection with my lifestyle to the tremendous discomfort my digestive problems left me with, nor did I consider my poor diet of fast food and processed foods contributing to this problem, not to mention bar food. In fact, I don't think I gave any consideration to the root cause; I just lived with it.

Finally, at age 37, I quit drinking, changed my eating habits, and gained direction and purpose. But, by this point, the damage was already well on its way. I went to chiropractic school, and there was a new kind of emotional stress in my life—studying, passing exams, and working very hard toward graduating with a Doctor of Chiropractic degree. I was a new Christian when I sold my house, quit my well-paying job, and moved hundreds of miles away from everyone I ever knew to go to school. It was hard acclimating to a new environment, living the Christian life in a very secular and even new-age culture. I found myself without the support of the believers I had related to before moving. My colitis flared up with a vengeance.

Stress plays a role in our physical, emotional, mental and spiritual health, and the challenges that can arise in these areas. Mental and emotional stress, chemical stress from the fast foods and alcohol I had consumed, the challenges of beginning a new journey in fulfilling my life's purpose, and trying to live a godly life as a new Christian impacted my overall health. Wholistic health involves considering the connections between stress i.e., mental/emotional, physical and chemical, and the physical body.

My childhood stresses and even traumas do not compare to that of many children today. The high number of extremely toxic vaccines kids receive before they even enter grade school, the toxic diet they are routinely fed at home as well as in school, and the lack of true social interaction with other kids as well as loving adults due to the high use of technology that continues to grow each year have heaped new and more damaging stressors than my generation could have imagined. Childhood trauma has increased exponentially, including physical, emotional, and sexual abuse as well as broken family homes and absentee parents.

This trauma results in a tremendous deficit in emotional health. The solutions to school violence and shootings are not merely greater gun control. The solution is to start taking back the true wholistic health of our children as well as the adults raising them. Poor wholistic health is a real problem that affects all of us.

Consider your underlying unhealthy emotional habits. How are they affecting your physical health, your spiritual health, your mental health? What are their root causes? What can you do to break these generational curses and follow a new path so you can lead your children, grandchildren, and those you influence in the direction of true health?

Some Emotional Health Statistics

Consider physical symptoms as well as the emotional, spiritual, and even mental symptoms as you read these statistics. Read them slowly and consider whether any of these apply to you or someone you know and love. Then ask yourself "what might the root be?" Pay close attention to the word "stress," as we will dig deeper into this word later in the book.

Top Causes of Stress in the United States:[4]

1. Job Pressure: Coworker Tension, Bosses, Work Overload
2. Money: Loss of Job, Reduced Retirement, Medical Expenses
3. Health: Health Crisis, Terminal or Chronic Illness
4. Relationships: Divorce, Death of Spouse, Arguments with Friends, Loneliness
5. Poor Nutrition: Inadequate Nutrition, Caffeine, Processed Foods, Refined Sugars
6. Media Overload: Television, Radio, Internet, E-Mail, Social Networking
7. Sleep Deprivation: Inability to Release Adrenaline and Other Stress Hormones

---

4 https://www.statista.com/topics/2099/stress-and-burnout/#topicOverview

Percent of People:[5]

Who say stress has a negative impact on their personal and professional life: 48%

Who say they have difficulty managing work and family responsibilities: 31%

Who reported being alienated from a friend or family member because of stress: 26%

People who cited physical symptoms (due to stress) experienced the following:[6]

Fatigue	51%
Headache	44%
Upset stomach	34%
Muscle tension	30%
Change in appetite	23%
Teeth grinding	17%
Change in sex drive	15%
Feeling dizzy	13%

People who cited psychological symptoms (due to stress) experienced the following:

Irritability or anger	50%
Feeling nervous	45%

5 Ibid

6 Ibid

Lack of energy	45%
Feeling as though you could cry	35%

Hopefully, after reading these, you can have a better appreciation of how our bodies are interconnected wholistically: how the emotional state of our health affects our physical, how our mental health affects our emotional and physical, and how this can impact our spiritual health and vice versa.

Hormones and Neurotransmitters

Every time someone tells me that they have been on antidepressants for years, my heart just breaks. I always wonder how thoroughly their brain chemicals—dopamine and serotonin particularly—have been assessed and monitored throughout those years. If that person has been under the care of conventional medicine, and I asked them how it was determined they were depressed, it's always been through subjective analysis, as with those treated for anxiety or any other mood disorder. It's subjective, meaning based on how the patient tells the doctor they feel. They *may* have had an initial basic blood serum test done on some basic hormones but nothing beyond that. No more follow up unless or until the patient adapts to the drug, and it is no longer working for them. Then, they simply take a different medication. Now my heart goes from broken to angry.

People are increasingly and routinely prescribed antidepressants without reevaluating the diagnosis or treatment through lab testing or looking for the root cause. This is a huge problem for Americans in particular.

For a brief time, I worked for another chiropractor when I first moved to North Carolina. My sole responsibility was to do new patient intakes and exams. Part of this process was to discuss their case history. I can't tell you how often patients listed antidepressants on their intake forms. I habitually asked if they were depressed. They consistently looked at me with a puzzled look on their face as if to say, "Why are you asking me that?" They would often answer in the negative. When I would pursue the questioning further by asking why they were taking an antidepressant and naming the drug they listed, they would then develop a look of understanding and explain that the doctor prescribed it to them because they had a hard time sleeping. They were on antidepressants for sleep!

Another common conversation is with people who have taken antidepressants for years. They refer to their health condition as chronic depression. First, I ask them how it was determined. They generally answer that it was based on how they feel—subjective. Then I ask if they have ever had a comprehensive neurotransmitter test done, they always look at me with a surprised look on their face, and I know the answer right away—they never knew this existed. As a side note, the best medium to check these brain chemicals is through saliva, and a combination of blood and saliva is even better.

If they have never had a proper assessment, nor follow up assessments, how does the practitioner even know what *all* the influencing neurotransmitters are or *if* that is truly the root cause of the problem? Diet is never taken into consideration and assessed, let alone other lifestyle factors, or toxic exposures to things like mold, heavy metals, pollutants, even electro-magnetic frequencies (EMF). The only component of their health that is considered before putting the patient on a highly addictive antidepressant, for life, is their emotional health.

The antidepressant drug market is a billion-dollar industry, and its leaders are aiming to grow rather than decrease this industry by reaching out to those who do not routinely seek care for their emotional health. As they do, biased assessments will continue, and drug sales will continue to increase.

The Connection between Our Hormones and Brain Chemicals

We really can't talk about our emotional health without sharing a little bit on how our hormones (e.g., estrogen, testosterone, and progesterone) and brain chemicals (e.g., dopamine, serotonin, GABA, acetylcholine, melatonin, leptin, and ghrelin), known as neurotransmitters, affect each other as well as our emotional health. Even appetite-regulating hormones can affect our overall health.

The subject of hormones and neurotransmitters is truly a complex and broad area, and there are hundreds of books dedicated to them alone. While I will not elaborate on each of these, it is important to develop an overall awareness of their function and influence on your health. Also, there is more to bringing each of them into balance than just taking a synthetic hormone or antidepressant.

You don't want to address the symptoms with a shot, patch, or pill because the symptoms can often point to the root cause of your physical health imbalances. Simply addressing symptoms or attempting to alter lab numbers could mask the root cause. It's also very possible that the hormone imbalance can be corrected when the root of a primary issue is resolved. They are very complex chemicals that are almost always misunderstood or overlooked entirely.

When people hear the word "hormones," they seem to limit their thinking to only reproductive hormones. However, there are far more hormones than our reproductive hormones. There are also hormones called neurotransmitters, regulated by electrical impulses sent throughout the nervous system. Other hormones (e.g., thyroid hormones, stress hormones, and reproductive hormones) are carried through the blood.

To address emotional health, this section will address the three primary reproductive hormones (i.e., estrogen, progesterone and testosterone) and neurotransmitters (i.e., serotonin, dopamine, GABA, and acetylcholine), exploring their function and how each directly influences emotional health.

All systems in the body are regulated by hormones and/or neurotransmitters. When your body is functioning optimally, you have even energy throughout the day; you sleep well at night; your emotions are within range of acceptable highs and lows, your menstrual cycle is regular; your sex-drive is healthy; you're maintaining a healthy weight; your hair, skin, and nails are healthy; your digestion is healthy; and your blood pressure, sugar levels, urinary function are functioning optimally. When they are not, hormones and/or neurotransmitters need to be taken into consideration as part of the full health assessment *before* determining a diagnosis, let alone before taking medications or undergoing hormone therapy.

Hormones

Cortisol is a hormone produced in the adrenal glands. The adrenals also release other hormones that have the responsibility of regulating blood sugar levels and regulating fluid pressure in the body. The adrenals release hormones called epinephrine and norepinephrine that signal other hormones in the brain called neurotransmitters to regulate their balances.

Cortisol helps the body physiologically deal with stress. When the body is stressed, it releases the hormone cortisol. Cortisol is also upstream of the chemical pathways in the body that regulate our reproductive hormones–estrogen, progesterone and testosterone.

When the body becomes chronically stressed, cortisol levels are disrupted and the other functions of the adrenal glands can be thrown out of balance, as well as the reproductive hormones downstream of the cortisol. The next section will more thoroughly address cortisol and the adrenal glands.

Estrogen stimulates the growth of tissue such as development of breast and reproductive organs and ensures their function.

In the brain, estrogen boosts the synthesis and function of neurotransmitters that affect sleep, mood, memory, libido, and cognitive factors such as learning and attention span.

Estrogen decreases the perception of pain, preserves bone mass, and increases HDL (i.e., good cholesterol). It also preserves the elasticity and moisture content of the skin, dilates blood vessels, and prevents plaque formation in blood vessel walls.

Progesterone is made primarily by the ovaries. The adrenal glands, peripheral nerves, and brain cells produce lesser amounts. Progesterone ensures the development and function of the breasts and female reproductive tract.

In the brain, progesterone binds to certain receptors to exert a calming, sedating effect. It improves sleep and protects against seizures.

Progesterone is also a diuretic. It enhances the sensitivity of the body to insulin and the function of the thyroid hormones. It contributes to bone growth and benefits the cardiovascular system by blocking plaque formation in the blood vessels and lowering the levels of triglycerides. Progesterone also can increase libido and contribute to the efficient use of fat as a source of energy.

Testosterone is manufactured by the ovaries in women, the testicles in men, and adrenal glands in both. It enhances libido and sexual response. It strengthens ligaments, builds muscle and bone, assists brain function, and is associated with assertive behavior and a sense of well-being. The level of testosterone influences both stamina and restful sleep. Testosterone has a protective effect against cardiovascular disease in men and women.

Each of these hormones affects our overall health in ways that extend beyond the function of reproduction. They also influence various functions of the brain. Obviously, if the reproductive hormones get thrown out of balance, they will influence the brain chemicals that affect our mood, energy, and sleep.

Depression is not simply treated with antidepressants prescribed quite possibly for the rest of a patient's life. Does it seem wise to do so without first testing the neurotransmitter levels, retesting as often as necessary? The solution is to get to the root cause of the emotional imbalances. This root cause could be emotional or physical trauma.

How do these hormones get thrown out of balance? The short answer is stress, including mental/emotional stresses; physical stresses; and chemical stresses like the air we breathe, the water we drink, and the foods we eat.

Keep in mind that cortisol responds to all stresses in the body and that cortisol is upstream in the chemical pathway of these reproductive hormones. The body will always respond to the demands of cortisol before worrying about the reproductive hormones being in balance.

Another reason could be that another organ or system of the body might be out of balance (e.g., cardiovascular health). There is a direct correlation between the gut and the brain. When there is inflammation in the gut, there is inflammation in the brain, potentially affecting our brain chemicals. The body works as a whole. It is not deficient in an antidepressant, anxiety medications, or sleep medications.

Uncovering the root cause and restoring the body to good balance is the true solution.

Neurotransmitters

Let's take a little deeper look at some of these brain chemicals to determine their primary functions, the potential consequences of imbalance, and their impact on our emotional and physical health.

Acetylcholine - This learning and memory neurotransmitter is the most important for conversion of short- to long-term memory.

Symptoms of Impaired Acetylcholine Activity:

- Loss of visual and photographic memory
- Loss of verbal memory
- Memory lapses
- Impaired creativity
- Diminished comprehension
- Difficulty calculating numbers
- Difficulty recognizing objects and faces
- Slowness of mental responsiveness
- Difficulty with directions and spatial orientation

Dopamine provides good feelings, pleasure, happiness, and satisfaction, even if they are temporary. This reward pathway produces good feelings in the brain and is related to repeating the action whenever possible.

Symptoms of Poor Dopamine Activity:

- Inability to self-motivate
- Inability to start or finish tasks
- Feelings of worthlessness
- Feelings of hopelessness
- Loss of temper for minor reasons
- Inability to handle stress
- Anger and aggression while under stress
- Desire to isolate oneself from others
- Unexplained lack of concern for family and friends

Signs Of Dopamine Imbalance:

- Iron-deficiency anemia
- Depression/lack of motivation
- Learning disorders and ADD
- Psychosis
- Schizophrenia
- Heavy menstrual cycles

Serotonin, Our Mood Booster - The primary function of serotonin is to stabilize your mood, as well as your feelings of happiness and well-being. Serotonin also plays a role in the digestive system and sleep cycles.

Symptoms of Impaired Serotonin Activity:

- Loss of pleasure in hobbies and interests
- Feelings of inner rage and anger
- Feelings of depression

- Difficulty finding joy from life pleasures
- Depression when it is cloudy or when there is lack of sunlight
- Loss of enthusiasm for favorite activities
- Not enjoying favorite foods
- Not enjoying friendships and relationships
- Unable to fall into deep restful sleep

GABA promotes feelings of calm, relaxation, social ease, and sleep.

Symptoms Associated with Gaba Imbalances:

- Feelings of anxiousness or panic for no reason
- Feelings of dread
- Feelings of inner tension and inner excitability
- Feelings of being overwhelmed for no reason
- Restless mind
- Hard to turn your mind off when you want to relax
- Disorganized attention
- Worry about things you never had thought of before

Tying it All Together

Now let's pull it together and see how both the hormones and neurotransmitters impact each other:

Hormones and Neurotransmitters (brain chemicals):

- Estrogen impacts serotonin in men and women
- Progesterone impacts GABA in men and women
- Estrogen impacts dopamine in women

- Estrogen impacts acetylcholine in women
- Testosterone impacts dopamine in men
- Testosterone impacts acetylcholine in men
- Thyroid hormone impacts all neurotransmitters receptors in men and women

Each of these hormones and brain chemicals are activated every time there is stress and trauma to the body, soul, and spirit. When they are chronically or traumatically challenged, a host of physical and emotional health problems can occur. This is also why it is so important that anyone who is stressed (and who isn't?) or has experienced trauma in their lives, sustains themselves on a healthy clean diet, gets proper sleep and exercise, drinks plenty of water to flush out the toxins (created by trauma and stress), and have their spines checked on a regular basis to assure good nerve supply.

Substances Commonly Recognized to Adversely Affect Our Hormones and Brain Chemicals

Our bodies were divinely made by our Creator to be adaptive and resilient. But over the years, as the industrial revolution developed and technology grew, we have come to learn how a lot of this progress has taken a toll on our physical bodies—most of the time unknown to us. While there has been some government regulation and oversight to protect us, there is probably as much, if not more, being approved regardless of the adverse effects to our health. Some of these assaults come from:

- **Industrial chemicals**: These chemicals are released into our air, our water, and in the working environment itself. Even at acceptable, government-regulated levels, these chemicals harm the nervous system and hormone levels over time, especially in children.

- **Pesticides**: These are used very heavily on all conventionally grown foods. Many are endocrine disruptors, throwing our hormones and brain chemicals way out of balance. When we consume conventionally raised foods, we are consuming these pesticides as well.
- **Prescription drugs** (the third-highest cause of neurotransmitter disease): If you consider the side effects of the antidepressants, anxiety medications, and other mood-altering medications, one of the (many) *common* side effects is often the symptom the medication was prescribed to relieve. In fact, almost all medications are like this. Start becoming familiar with the side effects of all medications and take these warnings seriously.
- **Abused drugs**: Any drug, including illegal drugs are going to adversely affect our emotional health as well as our physical health to an even far greater degree than prescription medications.
- **Food**: A more accurate way to state this is "food-like-substances." Approximately 85 percent of the foods we consume are chemically processed, genetically modified, and significantly altered from its original state. We consume so many toxic ingredients labeled as food, which also is void of the vital nutrients the body needs, including for our hormones and brain health.
- **Food additives**: Many of these artificial ingredients added to our food to make them last longer, look more colorful,

and taste sweeter are very toxic to the nervous system and very inflammatory.

- **Cosmetic ingredients**: Skin is the largest organ of the body but gets overlooked when it comes to protecting it from harmful ingredients. They are filled with toxic chemicals, a lot of them hormone disruptors, for the same reasons as food–preserving them, adding artificial colorings and even to taste better. What we put on our skin goes directly into the body.

Family, Community, and Connection

One more area that impacts our emotional health is connection with family, friends, and communities. God made us first for fellowship with Him and then with others. He also made us unique in every way, including our desire and tolerance to connect with others. Some folks are introverts, some are extroverts, and some (like me) are a mix of both. I often come off as an extrovert initially, but I do love alone time! I often say a good weekend for me is when my car never leaves the garage, the phone never rings, and I don't even communicate via text with anyone for days on end—this can be Heaven on Earth to me! Others can quickly fall into a state of feeling blue if they go one hour without some kind of social interaction. Most people also tend to change as they get older.

On the Appalachian Trail (AT), there is a phenomenon known as the "hiker bubble." Hikers who set out to complete the entire AT in 4–6 months typically start at the southern end of the Trail in Georgia around the beginning of March. Some may start a little sooner, others a little later. Some may start their hike at another point on the trail altogether then work their way back down to the beginning to finish later in the trek. But the group that starts at the beginning in March can be massive—several thousand hikers spread throughout a short period. And they basically move at the same pace, at least initially. Some will drop off sooner than later, others go faster, and others go slower. What happens next is this one big group breaks down into several smaller though still large groups. This is what is known as the hiker bubble.

That is way too many people for me! When I head for the mountains, I am heading for solitude. Not too long ago, we were sharing a campsite with a couple in their early forties. This young couple said they would love to go back and start their hike over again the following year, but this time follow a path that allowed them to connect with the hundreds of other people hiking at the same time! They were highly social and extroverts. While I enjoy connecting with people and do so quite easily, I truly need social rest after a time of heavy socializing—especially after attending a conference or something of that nature.

Connection and community are vital to our emotional health. This is where I know, especially as a single lady who does not have a husband, children, grandchildren, or even any family members who live close by, that I need to be intentional about connecting and building a community of like-minded folks. On the flip side, someone who is very social needs to have some self-awareness and bring themselves to a place of social rest from time to time. Because if you are not aware of either of these scenarios, your emotional health can become out of balance.

There are a variety of places one can build social connections. Family is one, of course. But if you don't have family close by, or if your family tends toward the dysfunctional side and it's not healthy for you to be around them for any length of time, there need to be alternatives.

One such alternative, whether your family unit is close or not, is the church family. It is vital to your emotional and spiritual health. I have weekly connections outside of church through my Toastmasters Club. I see these folks every week for an hour or so. We have a mutual interest in growing in our communication skills.

Another area can be those with like-minded hobbies. Mine is hiking and backpacking. Families and moms can connect with other families and moms. You can also connect at school or work. There are many places where social connections can be cultivated. Just like any good relationship, it takes work and commitment on the part of all.

Have social connections of all ages and cultures. When you leave this earth, no matter how old you may be, I pray that you have a church filled with people who have many personal stories of how they knew you, the influence you had on them, the love you showed them, and the many laughs you had together, celebrating your life in style! Can't you just feel the positive emotions from that kind of life? But it takes intentionality.

Solutions for Supporting Your Emotional Health

- For starters, pray. Be intentional about growing in your spiritual life. Get to personally know the God of the Universe, Jesus Christ, and the fruits of the Holy Spirit: peace, love, joy, kindness, goodness, faithfulness, and self-control—and ask for a fresh filling every morning.
- Find a Balance—Stop trying to fit 28 hours into a 24-hour day. This creates tremendous chronic emotional stress and

establishes poor discipline for adults as well as a poor model for children.

- Spend Time Outdoors—Just go outside into nature. Fresh air and sunshine do wonders for emotional health. You don't have to go far: it can be a local park or your backyard (if you're lucky enough to have one).
- Be Social—Connect with family, friends, church family, and community. For some this does not come naturally, so you need to be intentional about adding this component into your life.
- Create Work/Play Balance—This is especially important to do in your younger years so you don't burn yourself out by the time retirement rolls around.
- Take Care of Your Health—Care for your health as early and as much as you can, so you can enjoy your later years in good health.
- Seek Out God's Purpose for You— Live life with purpose. Have a reason to get out of bed in the morning and place a priority on your health.

Seek Necessary Professional Help

Explore the root cause of any emotional pain in the heart and heal from it. Abuse is trauma; it causes emotional and physical stress and can leave deep emotional wounds. Abuse of all kinds, on any level, is real, but you must develop the skills to manage your pain and forgive; otherwise the root of bitterness will eat you up from the inside out.

Call to Action: What are your underlying unhealthy emotional habits? How are they affecting your physical health, your spiritual health, your mental health? What are their root causes? What can you do to break these generational curses and follow on a new path so you can lead your children, grandchildren, and those you influence in the direction of true health?

True spiritual, mental, and emotional health really are in your control. I pray you believe these truths and start making steps toward receiving them. Begin by quieting yourself down, picturing yourself with Jesus, be open to spontaneous thought and vision and write down what you hear God telling you your purpose is in life. Ask Him about the first steps. Write them down in the form of goals and action steps. Don't just have a desire; be committed. Seek out emotional healing if needed. Taking charge of these areas of your health is not just empowering; it is true freedom.

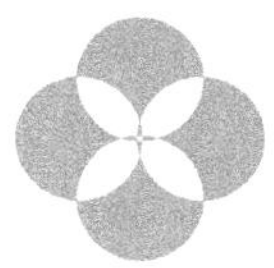

CHAPTER 5

Physical Health

"For you were bought with a price. So glorify God in your body."

—1 Corinthians 6:20 ESV

Over the years, as I worked with patients in my functional medicine practice, it became quite apparent to me that we are a "quick-fix" society. This is probably where my awareness and the material for my "Truth About Wellness" classes (and ultimately this book) originated. Did you know that in most, if not all, chronic degenerative disease conditions, the symptoms are the last thing to show up? Things brew beneath the surface—in most cases for many years—long before we are told something is wrong. In fact, any symptom—no matter how insignificant it may seem—is a sign that the body is out of balance. Don't ignore those messages from your body, especially if those symptoms persist or are constantly recurring. Your body is trying to tell you something is not right.

I am a retired chiropractic internist, not a pastor or psychiatrist. I have knowledge of the physical aspects of our health. Yet that doesn't exclude me from having discernment and objective unbiased common sense, nor should it exclude you. I realized quickly that I couldn't fix everything and everyone. Sometimes, the root of a patient's problem isn't physical but rather lies in another part of the health pie (e.g., mental, emotional, or even spiritual). But I also learned quickly that in my specialty, physical health, I needed to first start with the foundational basics with my patients, taking it one step at a time. If we did not first address the five foundational components that make up the physical health quadrant (i.e., rest, water, exercise, good nutrition, and good nerve supply), we would be swimming upstream and causing great frustration for both my patient and me. If we did not start with these basics and create solid discipline within each of these areas first, it would also be a very costly battle in time and money for the patient as well.

Let's dive a little deeper into these five components of the physical quadrant so you can have a greater appreciation of the vitalness of each, and the roles they play, not only in restoring our bodies back to good physical health but also bringing greater balance to our mental, emotional, and spiritual selves.

The Truth about Rest

I encounter people daily who tell me they don't have enough energy and want to know what medications they can take. First, if you are one of these people, and your objective is to restore your body back to good health using natural approaches, this is the wrong question to ask. You should be asking yourself "what is the *root cause* of why I don't have energy?" Not "what can I take?"

The first question I ask is about their quantity and quality of sleep: You won't have energy if you are not sleeping enough and/or sleeping well.

The only time the body can heal and repair itself (e.g., build new cells) is when it is sleeping. The body does its best healing and repairing between 10:00 p.m. and 12:00 a.m. If you are not *asleep* between these hours, not just in bed, you have just lost the most essential time for your body to heal and repair. There's a reason that so many of our ancestors followed the cycles of the sun and the moon. We truly should be in sync with the cycles of the sun and the moon rising and setting. In winter, when the days are shorter, we could really be asleep even earlier.

Lack of quality sleep has a direct negative impact on most chronic degenerative diseases. If you are not getting your proper sleep, it stresses the adrenal glands, two triangular glands that sit one on top of each kidney. They perform a whole lot of vital functions. Previous sections addressed some of those functions when discussing emotional health, and the next section will examine their importance.

But let's recap for now. One of the main things the adrenals do is release a hormone called cortisol, which is the body's natural anti-inflammatory. It responds to all stresses to the body—mental/emotional stress, chemical stress, and physical stress. Lack of sleep is a physical stress to the body.

It's a cyclical problem; if we don't give our bodies enough rest, our adrenal glands can't perform properly, and if our adrenal glands aren't performing properly, we might not be sleeping well. We also might have blood sugar imbalances, blood pressure issues, reproductive hormone problems, thyroid challenges, and/or emotional issues—all of which the adrenals influence.

So, what can you do? For starters, remove the TV and computer from the bedroom. Stop watching TV or using the computer—including cell phones—30 minutes before you want to be asleep. Plan to be *asleep* no later than 10:00 p.m. Sleep for at least seven hours—nine is better. Remove the biggest offenders that stress the adrenal glands. Cigarettes are the leading toxin you could introduce to your body. In second place is diet soda, and a close third is regular soda. We will talk more about food choices that also stress the adrenals in the next chapter.

Perhaps you are a "night owl" and can't fathom falling asleep until well after midnight and not rising until well after the sun does. If so, I suggest setting an alarm clock for just 30 minutes earlier than you normally get up. Place it across the room so you must get out of bed to turn it off—and then stay up once you are out of it! Continue to set the alarm earlier and earlier until you are conditioned to arise within the seven- to nine-hour window from the proper and healthier time you went to sleep. Also, turn the temperature down at night—a cooler room is much better for the body to fall asleep. If possible, use a thermostat with a timer to start warming your room or house up a bit come morning.

Supplement with a *quality* melatonin (*not* something you would get at a discount department store, drug store, or dollar store), along with a calming herb like ashwagandha, lemon balm, valerian root, holy basil, or theanine. If you are prescribed sleeping medications, antidepressants, or any other medications, check with your pharmacist first to see if there could possibly be any drug interactions.

Take the time to observe why you can't fall or stay asleep. Consider your diet when it is closer to bedtime; are you consuming caffeine, especially in the form of chocolate? Try to adjust your habit to eliminate caffeinated drinks and foods right before going to bed. Is your mind racing about the things you need to do the next day? Try putting a little notebook by your bed to jot those thoughts down, get them out of your head, and deal with them in the morning. All these things combined can help make for a much better night's sleep for you.

Water, Water, Water: The Truth about Water!

Water is literally vital to the health of every cell in our bodies. Picture a very dry, cracked Arizona desert. The land has not seen rain in months; then the monsoon hits. During the first hour of rain, the ground is so dry that the water just runs off. After a few hours of constant watering, the land gets wet and then saturated, allowing the water to seep deep into the soil. Or picture a dried-up sponge on the back of your sink. You try to mop up some spilled liquid, but the sponge is so dry it's almost worthless. But if you were to wet that sponge, wring out the excess, and then mop up the liquid, it does a good job absorbing the water. Now think of that desert land or that sponge as each individual cell in your body. Are your cells saturated with water as they need to be, or are they dry and parched, crying out for help before they die?

Do you have constipation, headaches, joint or muscle pain, dry hair, or dry skin? Maybe you don't like the taste of water. These and many other signs could be an indication that your body is dehydrated, which starts way before you are thirsty. In fact, people who say they can go all day without drinking any water are very likely dehydrated. Water is *vital* to life!

There are four main organs or systems that the body uses to rid its waste and toxins. Fifty percent of the body's waste *should* be eliminated through the kidneys. Twenty-five percent should be eliminated through the skin, twenty-three percent through the lungs, and two percent through the colon. These four mechanisms, however, must have *water* for the waste and toxins to come out of the body. And the only way the body can get water is if *you* provide it!

We do get some of our water from fruits and vegetables—that is, if you are eating fruits and vegetables. While a little bit can come from the air we breathe, the rest must come from us literally drinking pure, fresh, wet water—and lots of it. I'm not talking about "liquids" that have water in them; tea and coffee do not count. When I ask patients and customers if they drink enough water, they vehemently say "yes!" until I tell them how much we need to drink each day. At a minimum, we need half of our body weight in ounces of water per day. For example, if a person weighs 150 pounds, they need to drink 75 ounces of water per day. If you are drinking coffee or other caffeinated drinks, you need to replenish an equal amount of water in addition to your minimum, as caffeine dehydrates. If you are sweating from exercise, or working out in the heat, you need to replenish the amount you've lost in sweat as well. To most people, this is a *lot* of water, but this is the truth—that is how dehydrated we really are.

When I suggest not drinking soda, milk and sports drinks, people generally respond (with despair in their voice) "then what can I drink?!" My answer is always "water!" Our bodies truly do not need any other liquid but water. When we drink water, it's like giving our bodies a bath on the inside—it's cleansing! However, if you do not drink enough water, the toxins and waste stay inside of you, causing inflammation in the body, which then leads to many sicknesses and disease. Dehydration causes a lower state of health.

Two cautionary notes: first, don't ever drink water or anything liquid with your meals. This dilutes your digestive enzymes which are needed to break your food down. Second, don't drink municipal tap water if you can help it. It contains chlorine and, in a lot of cases, fluoride which, contrary to popular belief, is not good for you. It interferes with the function of the thyroid, along with contributing to a cascade of other problems. If you are on well water, make sure it is tested for any heavy metals.

Some facts about water:

- Water makes up 75 to 80 percent of your body's cells.
- Water supplies oxygen to the tissues (think H2O—the "O" is the oxygen).
- Water is used by the body for digestion, circulation, absorption, elimination, lubrication, and temperature control.
- Eight to ten glasses of water per day could help ease back and joint pain.
- Tap water contains impurities that become toxins in the body.
- Lack of water equals lack of oxygen.
- Lack of oxygen could be a leading cause of why people are tired.
- Parasites, viruses, and bacteria are anaerobic, which means they survive without oxygen!
- By the time you are thirsty, you are already dehydrated!

Start gradually and increase the amount of water you drink every few days. Carry a water bottle everywhere you go. Know how many ounces it holds and determine how many bottles you need to drink each day to reach your minimum. Spread your intake throughout the day. Drink more in the earlier part of the day so you won't wake up in the middle of the night to use the bathroom.

Initially, you'll probably find yourself needing the restroom quite frequently at first, but gradually, as your body gets rehydrated (and this can take several months), your frequency will decrease. Remember the dry parched desert? It's kind of like heavy rain hitting the ground after a long drought—the water just runs off. Eventually, it starts saturating the ground and staying in. Relish each time you urinate or sweat or have a good bowel movement because toxins are coming out of your body rather than staying in and polluting it.

The Types of Water

I'd like to tell you a personal story about my own experience with water. There is a *difference* regarding the *type* of water we drink. But before I continue, I'd like to caution you to not get all hung up on what type for now, especially if you are not drinking any water at all—for starters, well, just start!

While I was practicing in Charleston, South Carolina, a sales rep for a particular water- filtering machine came into my office and asked to give me a water demonstration of his product. He first demonstrated to me the acidity versus the alkalinity pH of various drinks, including some brands of bottled water. He had soda, coffee, an energy drink, tap water, and several brands of bottled water. The objective, of course, is to drink more alkalizing water; we don't want to consume too many acidic liquids or foods. Everything he tested, using simple pH strips, was all on the scale of acidity, from very acidic to the tap water being neutral (a 7 on the pH scale).

Even some brands of the bottled water were slightly acidic. Then he showed me the pH of the water that came from his water machine: alkalizing! I believe it was a 10.

He then demonstrated the absorbability of the waters using tea bags, which were representative of the cells' ability to take in the various liquids. Once again, the machine he was demonstrating showed the highest absorbability.

The third factor he demonstrated was the water's oxygen reduction potential (ORP)—that is the ability to fight off free radicals, the things that cause cancer. He used a device called an ORP meter. Of course, the water filtration machine fared best.

Although I told him I trusted and believed his demonstration, I was most interested in what *my* body needed, whether it was a higher pH water or nothing—if my cells were already absorbing water efficiently.

He offered to let me try the water for a whole month. He would bring me gallons of water, as much as I wanted or needed, if I didn't drink anything else. I agreed.

There were several measuring sticks I was going to use for myself. At the time, I was drinking nothing but reverse osmosis water that I would get from a machine at my local big-box store. Reverse osmosis water, I later learned, is not the best form of water to drink. It is void of any of the natural healthy minerals that are vital to our body—magnesium, sodium, and potassium.

I was training for a marathon that year, in the mid-summer Charleston heat, and at the same time I was also going through menopause. Both were drawing on my adrenals more than normal. I had absolutely no energy. Where just in the previous year I could jog six miles in an hour in the mid-day summer heat, I was now having to slow down to a walk about every five minutes. This was one measuring stick I was going to use.

The other measuring stick was a test I used to run on myself (as well as my patients) called a Body Chemistry Diagnostic test. I loved this test; unfortunately, the maker of this product has since closed his business. Several of the markers it checked that were out of balance for me (and getting worse) were oxidative stress (i.e., the body's ability to fight off free radicals) and electrolytes e.g., magnesium, sodium, potassium. My oxidative stress numbers continued to climb higher each time I checked it, and my electrolytes continued to get lower. Both measures were drastically high and low, respectively. No matter what I did (e.g., eating well, exercising, drinking water), there was no improvement to these markers.

I remained faithful for the whole month, not changing anything else but the water I was drinking. Truthfully, in less than a week's time I noticed an actual improvement in my running ability. I am not such a sensitive person that I can notice a magical difference because of anything I normally do to take care of my health—at least not in the short run, including my chiropractic adjustments (although I know they make a difference). This was quite remarkable for me!

At the end of the months' time, I ran the Body Chemistry Diagnostics test again and—lo and behold—there was improvement! For the first time in about nine months, I saw improvement to each of the markers that had been getting worse for me. However, at the time, I was unable to afford this brand of water ionizer machine; since it was a multilevel marketing product, the price was higher than some others that were not part of this sales model.

After researching other brands, I eventually was able to buy a Tyent water ionizer. There are other comparable brands out there as well. Truly, *anything* is better than regular tap water. If a water ionizer is out of your budget, I recommend drinking bottled *spring* water, which retains minerals. Don't drink distilled water or reverse osmosis water unless you are doing a short temporary fast or detox or something similar. Regarding the brand of bottled water to buy, I recommend buying some pH strips (they are quite inexpensive) and doing your own testing to see which brand fares best. There are also "smart" waters and other types of water that report having a high pH. They are typically higher in price, and so I would do the same: test them for yourself to see if what they claim is true and which one is best. Filters like Brita are another option if budget is a concern. What is still on my wish list is a whole-house water filter system—this would cover everything from the water I drank, cooked in, cleaned with, and bathed with.

After this experience, I became a firm believer in quality water. However, if tap water is your only option, by all means, it's still a better choice than anything else you could possibly be drinking—far better. Now, go drink some water!

The Truth about Exercise

I'm going to take a chance here and first share the good news with those of you who despise exercising—but only if you promise me you will continue to read beyond what I'm getting ready to say and grab hold of the "really good news!" Ready? Over-exercising can be a physical stress to the body. There, I said it—but don't use this as an excuse to not exercise! Remember: everything in balance. Not exercising also contributes to stress in the body. Now for the really good news.

I can tell you from personal experience the importance and value of exercise. Wintertime is admittedly harder for me to get out and jog like I enjoy doing because it's too cold for this very thin-blooded girl! And I see it on the scale too, which proves to me that without exercise I will not see the results in my health as I would like. I also know I'm like a bear in winter—I will come out of my hibernation in springtime and start my outdoor activities again like jogging and backpacking and my metabolism will reset to a faster pace. However, as the years go by, I find that this entire process takes a little longer each year for me. Our metabolism slows as we age; it's just a matter of how healthy we are that determines how quickly or slowly this will take place.

Exercise is so important for many reasons. We know it's important for our cardiovascular health; it strengthens the heart muscles and gets the blood pumping strong and lungs working fully.

Exercise is a *great* stress reliever! Who doesn't need *that* these days? Some days I am like the character Forrest Gump. Stress is my fuel, and when it is topped off to the max, I could just keep running until that fuel is emptied out and I feel relaxed again. It works wonders! Even traditional medicine practitioners say exercise is a more effective remedy for depression than an antidepressant.

Our lymphatic system is like the sewage system of our bodies. The body's waste travels through the lymph system before being dumped into the liver to get sorted out for elimination. However, the only way this waste can travel through the lymph vessels is by our arms, legs, heart, lungs, and other muscles pumping it out. The muscles can only pump if we use and exercise them. Otherwise, our "sewage system" becomes sluggish, and the "garbage" stays in us instead of moving out, causing us to become toxic, which leads to inflammation and disease.

When we exercise it causes us to sweat. Remember, 25 percent of our body's waste is eliminated through the skin, primarily through perspiration. Sweating is good! I think some people, women in particular, have an aversion to exercise because they either consciously, or perhaps subconsciously, don't want or like to sweat. Twenty-three percent of our body's waste should be eliminated through the lungs. Exercise gets the bad air out (carbon dioxide) and gets the fresh, good air in (oxygen), working the muscles of the lungs. Otherwise, those toxins stay *inside* the body, which is not good.

I know that right about now some of you are saying, "but I hate to exercise!" And I'm saying, "but read what I just said!" It is vital to your health to exercise, and there are many ways to accomplish this. Let me pause here to say that vacuuming the house or lifting things at your job is not "exercise"—it's work! Unless you are consistently performing these tasks at a steady heart rate for 20—30 minutes. If you clean a house at that pace, I would love to hire you! Of course, you burn calories doing these things, but to benefit your health, it takes more. We really should be exercising a minimum of three times per week for at least 20—30 minutes each time. That way, you get the heart muscles pumping, the lungs expanding, and the sweat coming out.

Here Are Some Health Facts on Exercising:

- The fuel that powers your body is sugar/glucose.
- Muscles store glucose in the muscle fibers.
- Muscles can't store much glucose, so they signal the body for more fuel.

- When the glucose supply is gone, the body starts breaking down fat molecules into fuel.
- Fat molecules have more energy than glucose molecules.
- The process of breaking down fat requires oxygen.
- Lack of oxygen for fat breakdown will result in lactic acid buildup.
- Aerobic exercise also exercises the arteries and strengthens the artery walls.
- Strong arteries allow for less cholesterol buildup.
- Diets high in "bad" fats, sugars, and starches plus a sedentary lifestyle leads to diabetes!
- Bodies also convert glucose into fat.
- Moderate exercise more than doubles the rate at which your lymph circulates; the faster the white blood cells circulate, the more cancer cells and viruses they can pick off and the stronger your immune system becomes!

We have so many exercise options to choose from in my town, and I have a feeling there are in yours as well. There are quite a few fitness centers around if you like traditional exercise such as cardio-vascular machines, weights, and aerobics classes. Here in western North Carolina, we also have a huge playground right in our own backyard called the mountains! I backpack, and there is nothing like heading off to the mountains and breathing in the refreshing crisp air, far from the noises of life while taking in the beauty of God's creation all around me! Talk about decompressing and enhancing your health—wow! And you know what? It's *free*!

Many towns, cities, and even more rural areas have greenways or rails to trails for their community members to enjoy and benefit from; look for one close to your area—you might be surprised what you will find! Even if you live in a city, you can go out and exercise along the streets before the workday begins or on weekends. Or "borrow" someone else's neighborhood if yours is not inviting. When I lived in Charleston, I loved to go downtown early in the morning, especially on weekends, and just enjoy the beauty of the historic city while I jogged. I'd then treat myself to a cup of cappuccino at a little sidewalk café as my reward! Your county Parks & Recreation website, the local Chamber of Commerce, and Visitor Bureau will most likely have a wealth of enjoyable opportunities for you too.

Take an Exercise Inventory to Get You Started

1. Ask yourself: What is exercise to you?
2. What might keep you from exercising—time, location, dislike, etc.?
3. How can you overcome these barriers?
4. Are you currently on a REGULAR exercise program?
5. How often do you exercise?
6. For how long?
7. What kind of exercise are you doing?
8. What might you think are the benefits of exercise to you?

It's time to get out and start power walking, join a fitness center, hike a mountain, and become *alive*!

Good Nerve Supply: What *Is* It and Why You Should Care?

When you hear the word "chiropractor" what is the first thing you think of? Back or neck pain? Well, here is another "truth" for you: that is *not* what chiropractic care is all about. When you hear the phrase "good nerve supply" what do you think of? You probably have never heard it before, have you? How about the word "subluxation?" Well, let me take a few minutes and explain to you about another foundational piece of the physical health quadrant.

Subluxation is a word you probably have never heard before unless you have been to a chiropractor. In a very simple sense, subluxation is when the bones in our back or neck, called vertebra, are misaligned. Just a millimeter of shift is all it takes, and they can stay stuck or locked in that position, putting pressure on the spinal nerves that pass in between the bones. Initially, you most likely won't even feel the pressure but it causes a lower state of health for us. These nerves are the roots of the entire communication highway from the brain to the body and back up again—they are *very* important! Every cell, tissue, organ, and system of the body needs good nerve supply.

Quite often this pressure is not being felt, even in the back or neck. In fact, back and neck pain are just two of the many symptoms that are a result of nerve interference. The misalignment I am talking about isn't a gross dislocation; just a millimeter of shift is enough to put pressure on the spinal nerves. Equivalent to the weight of a single dime, this pressure can decrease communication from the brain to the body by 40 percent! This is like stepping on the hose when we are trying to water the garden—without enough water, it won't grow and be nourished properly, and it might die. The same is true for the cells, tissues, organs, and systems in our body. If they don't get the proper nerve supply, they will not function optimally, and in fact, they could die—especially if left uncorrected for any length of time. You would likely never try to run your computer at 60 percent capacity. How much more important is your body?

Many things can cause subluxations, such as poor posture; poor sleeping habits; repetitive motions; injuring ourselves at work, home, or play; automobile accidents; and even the birthing process. Remember, a lot of the time—in fact most of the time—we are not even feeling these subluxations early on. Then the forces and stresses of life keep impacting that subluxated area of the spine until eventually we realize a lower state of health.

Every function of the body requires nerve supply, and that function will be adversely affected when there is nerve interference. Each spinal nerve is like the trunk of a tree; they keep branching and branching clear down to a cellular level. Interference to one nerve root has an impact on many areas of the body—and there is almost always more than one nerve root compromised within a person's spine at any given time. If you are experiencing a lower state of health in any capacity and are working toward restoring the body back to good health, restoring good nerve supply needs to be included in your health plan.

We all should have our spines checked on a regular basis throughout our lives. Just as we should be eating properly and exercising throughout life to achieve and maintain optimum health, so must we maintain the health of our spine.

Don't overlook this vital aspect of your health regime; make an appointment with a chiropractor today. As with every other expert or professional, chiropractors too have different philosophies and objectives. Here are a couple of differences:

Pain Relief versus Correction

There are three basic schools of thought when it comes to chiropractic philosophies: wellness care, pain-based care, and functional chiropractic. One school of thought is what is known as "straight" chiropractic. In the purest sense, this philosophy believes that the chiropractor's sole responsibility is to adjust the spine, freeing up nerve interference, and allowing the body to heal itself. This philosophy basically abides by the "getting to the root cause" philosophy. However, straight chiropractors think that the root cause of all health problems is always subluxations to the spine. While they consider whether the patient is dehydrated, malnourished, or stressed, they do not feel it is their professional responsibility to guide you in a better direction in these areas. This philosophy believes in maintaining the health of your spine for a lifetime, and I agree whole-heartedly. The college I attended, Sherman College of Chiropractic, falls under this philosophy. Originally known as Sherman College of Straight Chiropractic, this institution dropped the "straight" designation a few years ago, while retaining the same philosophy. Insurance coverage under this wellness chiropractic care usually is not available. Most of the time pain drives a patient to seek treatment; if it is "acute" then insurance may cover it at least for the short term.

The other end of the spectrum to this philosophy is what is known as pain based or "mixer" chiropractic. This is what you will see more of—at least when you look at their yellow page ads or nowadays, the websites for a lot of chiropractors. In my opinion, they are primarily chasing after what the insurance companies allow—addressing acute pain. They may incorporate therapies such as electric muscle stimulation, intersegmental traction, and heat and ice therapy to help with the symptoms. Once you are out of pain (or you have met the max your insurance will allow) your treatment is done until the next time you are in pain. Meanwhile, your spine continues to degenerate because it's not being maintained. Insurance will most likely cover this type of treatment because it's primarily "acute" care.

There is a hybrid philosophy that tends to lean more toward the straight chiropractic, yet the chiropractor is much more wholistic and functions in the true capacity of a primary care doctor who only uses natural approaches. This is what I call a functional chiropractor. I was introduced to this philosophy a couple years into my practice, and ultimately received my diplomat in internal disorders, and became board certified as a chiropractic internist.

It's not well known, but depending on each state's licensing law, some chiropractors are licensed to do pelvic and prostate exams and even deliver babies. Others are licensed to do intravenous nutrition therapy and chelation (i.e., removing certain heavy metals from the bloodstream). In most states, chiropractors can order and interpret blood work and other specialty labs, and in some, chiropractors can do the blood draws themselves. Personally, this is the type of chiropractor I would encourage you to seek, as they can do both: address your spinal health and act in the capacity as a primary care provider. If you already have a functional medicine doctor, then look to a "straight" chiropractor to maintain your spine, or at least a mixer chiropractor who is willing to set you up on a wellness plan to maintain the health of your spine.

Who Can Benefit from Chiropractic Care?

The answer is everyone! Anyone who has a spine and is breathing—from cradle to grave, from the first day to the last day of life. In fact, there are even animal chiropractors—I know cats, dogs, horses, and a slew of other animals have benefited from chiropractic care as they too have a nervous system and vertebra that can become subluxated.

Remember, it's not about pain, but rather about removing nerve interference. Of course, the techniques that are used for a day-old baby or an 80-year-old osteoporotic woman would be different from how a chiropractor would adjust a full-grown healthy adult. Everyone truly should have their spines routinely checked and maintained throughout life. I personally have consistently received routine chiropractic care for almost 30 years now. With a few exceptions, I have gone to my chiropractor every 2 weeks during that time. I have lived in six different towns over those years, and one of the first things I did when I moved each time was to find a chiropractor who was in line with my wholistic philosophy.

The Truth about the Foods That Heal and the Foods That Kill

We are what we eat! The saying should also include "and what we drink too." It's a wonder I don't look like a convenience store burrito with extra cheese, given how many of those late-night snacks I had in my before-Jesus days! Thank God He can restore not only souls but bodies as well! Before I came to learn the truth about wellness, my diet was horrible. I was a walking example that just because you are thin doesn't mean you have a healthy diet or a healthy body.

At the beginning of the book, we talked about making a new paradigm shift in our thinking. I would like to ask you to give thought to making a new paradigm shift in how to determine what foods to eat. We have been wrongly told what foods to eat and not to eat for so long—especially by our government, the corporate food industry, as well as television ads, magazine articles, colleagues, friends, family, the latest diet fad, and anyone else who thinks they know. To top it off, it seems like this information changes every couple of years "eat this, no don't eat that." There are so many diets and opinions out there our heads can spin like a crazy top. Just keep it all on a shelf for a while longer, or at least through the end of the book. It's time to shift this paradigm to the truth as well. Reflect on the current paradigm of what you've been told healthy eating is and how that has been working for you. I recognize some may say "fine." And that's okay—but I'm talking to those of you who are tired of the up and down roller coaster of dieting, while at the same time continuing to see your health decline. I think this latter group outnumbers those who say their eating is "fine."

So here is the first key to the new paradigm: it's not about the calories! I know, I know—that's what we've always been taught. It's also not about the fat grams, carbohydrates, proteins, or salt, portion sizes, or the number of "points." Don't get me wrong; these are important, and our bodies need all of these in the right form. But these should not be our measuring stick as to the foods we choose to eat. Again, let me ask you how that has been working for us? It hasn't! Just look around you—look at your coworkers, the schools (scary), your church family, your own family, your fellow shoppers—the grocery store, a discount department store (really scary!), the obese person sitting in the car next to you munching on a processed sandwich they just picked up from the drive-through window that was listed as "low calorie" on the menu board. It's not working for us. As a society, we are sicker and more overweight than ever before. Okay, okay: I'll get off my soapbox (for the moment!) and tell you what it is about.

Eating well is about consuming the right *nutrients*. We should not be eating to be *full*; rather, we should eat to be *nourished*. As much as we eat, and as overweight as many people are, we are still a very malnourished society. This leads to chronic degenerative diseases like diabetes, heart disease, high cholesterol, depression, thyroid problems, obesity, autoimmune diseases, and yes, even (and especially) cancer. The list goes on and on.

I saw a meme once that said, "*90 calories sells a lot better than 30 ingredients. Convincing the world to count calories instead of ingredients is one of the most profitable schemes ever.*" I couldn't have said this better myself. I would like to add counting calories instead of counting *nutrients* is where we have been greatly deceived, at the expense of our health, and even our lives.

Let's now take a greater look at more of these deceptions and how to overcome them.

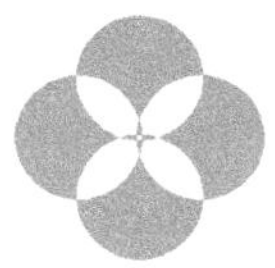

CHAPTER 6

Inflammatory versus Noninflammatory Foods

"And God said, "Behold, I have given you every plant yielding seed that is on the face of all the earth, and every tree with seed in its fruit. You shall have them for food."

—Genesis 1:29 ESV

I can't even begin to count, or even imagine how many "weight loss diets" have come and gone throughout the past century or more. Much information has come down the pike, mostly from our government, the medical world, and the food industry, over those same years, telling us one year *this* is bad for us, and the next year *that* is old information, now *this* is bad for us. In the meantime, our population has become sicker and sicker. The United States spends the most amount of money on "healthcare" than any other industrialized country, and yet we have the sickest population of people. As of 2024, 54 percent of children in the United States are chronically ill. This is our next generation starting off their adult life behind the eight ball.

A better measuring stick to determine which foods to avoid and which to eat is whether those foods are inflammatory or noninflammatory. Inflammation is at the root of all chronic diseases. It stands to reason, then, that we should avoid foods that cause inflammation in the body.

Let's break these down by what I call the "short list" of inflammatory foods (i.e., acidic pH foods) and the short list of noninflammatory foods (i.e., alkalizing pH foods). These short lists are to hopefully help simplify things for you when you are planning your menu for the week, grocery shopping, dining out, or having a meal at a friend's home. This also helps keep our food choices more general. Everybody is different, their bodies are different, there is no magic diet (and there are many out there!) that works for everyone. But a great place to start, that will go a long way in restoring yours and your children's health, or maintaining it, is to avoid some common foods that cause inflammation. And it would behoove us to consume as many non-inflammatory foods, which also convert into nutritious foods, as much as possible. Remember, we are what we eat.

Let's start with the inflammatory foods, the foods that are literally killing us. I will elaborate on the noninflammatory foods in a minute, but for now, I encourage you to use each of these lists as your new filter when trying to determine if a food is healing or killing you.

Inflammatory Foods

- Fast Food

- Fried Foods
- PACKAGED and PROCESSED foods (this list of foods is huge)
- Sugars
- Animal Products
- Grains

These last two are real foods, and can be eaten, but I will explain in a little bit the safe way to eat these foods. The first four however, aren't even *real* foods; they are "food-like substances." These foods have no nutritional value; in fact, they are literally killing us.

Now let's break each of these inflammatory foods down a little more.

The Truth about Fast Foods

I grew up in Johnstown, Pennsylvania—a small rural town in the southwestern part of the state, about two hours east of Pittsburgh. At some point in the 1960s, the first McDonald's restaurant opened in Johnstown. I can remember going there as a treat for Sunday lunches. Unlike a lot of American families in the 1960s, Sunday was the only day my stay-at-home mom of five kids *didn't* cook. This McDonald's was a walk-up window, and we would bring our delightful hamburgers home to sit down and eat. I can still remember the wrapping paper they came in (white for plain burgers, yellow paper for cheeseburgers), and the little paper sleeve that the fries came in. We typically did not have soda in the house, but most likely, we had soda with our McDonald's meals too. *Or* a milkshake—chocolate for me, please! But today? Sadly, today, fast-food options are a mainstay of the American diet, any day of the week.

Most of us know that eating fast food and fried food is unhealthy—after all, we've been hearing that for years—and I won't argue with that. Some people think those foods are off-limits only if they want to lose weight; otherwise, they still eat them. Or they choose a meal with "low calories" thinking they made a healthy choice. These are favorite foods of children and teenagers alike. It's also a favorite go-to for busy adults, especially moms and dads who are juggling working outside the home and parenting at the same time. But please, please hear me: These food-like substances are KILLING you AND your children. Foods that were once a "treat" have become the staple for American families, and make no mistake, they are a root cause of many health problems these days, especially for our children.

Did you know that at least one popular fast-food burger joint puts sugar in their salt for the French fries to make you come back for more? It works, trust me I've been there. These places haven't stayed in business for over 80 years because they are cheap and fast—the former not even being the case these days. They have top scientists working on their foods to entice your palate to keep coming back for more.

The Truth about Fried Foods

Who doesn't love salty and crunchy foods, or something so sweet almost to the point of being sickening? What draws any one of us to these heavenly fried foods? I can just walk by a restaurant and smell the food cooking inside and I salivate. How about a county fair—oh boy, look out! What is the common denominator of all these stimulators? Trans fats, that's what. "What is wrong with that," you might ask. It literally is our death sentence, especially if consumed on a chronic basis. Trans fats are what give foods the crunch and even the mouth feel. Bet you never thought about "mouth feel" before, have you?

These foods are very, very inflammatory. They are processed to the point that they are no longer real food. All the nutrients have been cooked out of them. Not only that, but toxic substances have taken their place. Trans fats—right up there with sugars—are some of the most toxic substances you can put into your body. While they might satisfy that addictive craving in the moment, every bite is another nail in the coffin, so to speak. Eaten chronically, they literally will shorten your lifespan. Leading food scientists work for the companies that make these foods. They diligently study *your* "tipping point"—that point where you wouldn't take another bite, and they back down by one notch. They know how to keep you coming back for more; it's called "addiction." Yes, there is intentionality to make people become (quickly) addicted to these foods. Remember the potato chip slogan "bet you can't eat just one"? They weren't kidding; they were telling you ahead of your putting your hand into that bag what they were setting out to do to you. You just had to take their bait, their challenge—and you lose.

Another truth about all foods that are not healthy for us—not just fried foods and trans fats—is we cannot "exercise" them away. It's important to remember we are not talking calories here; we are talking nutrients versus toxins.

Just like anything else inflammatory, when we consume fried and trans-fatty foods, it triggers a cascade of chemical reactions in the body that ultimately end up causing inflammation. This affects not just your vasculature, but also your sinuses, gut, joints, brain, skin—everywhere. It also disrupts other vital functions in the body such as when the adrenal glands must release cortisol to address that inflammation. Our reproductive hormones, brain chemicals (called neurotransmitters), fluid levels regulated by the kidneys (including our blood pressure), and our sugar levels are all disrupted. These toxic foods bog down the functions of our liver—a vital organ that we will talk more about in the next section. Eating fried/trans fatty foods as well as the multitude of other foods that cause inflammation can lead to diabetes, depression, anxiety, hypertension, cardiovascular disease, arthritis, and reproductive issues, just to name a few!

Right about now there are likely some of you who are puffing out your chests, noses turned up, a slight tone of pride in your voices saying, "I never eat *those* foods." Maybe so, but there is another type of food that is killing us just as quickly: packaged and/or processed foods. Do you eat those? Before you say "no" let me tell you what these foods are.

The Truth about Packaged and Processed Foods

Let's now delve a little deeper to learn how to determine if a packaged food is okay to eat, as well as the *real* foods we need to be wary of, and the foods that can be our medicine.

Anything that has a food label on it and comes in a package is a "packaged food." Yes, this includes any hot or cold cereal, bread (including wheat bread), lunchmeat (also a processed food), bacon, dairy products (including yogurts), canned soups and vegetables, chips, frozen foods, toaster pastries, pizza, soda (the worst!)—the list goes on and on.

The food industry has done a tremendous job in deceiving us to believe that these foods are "healthy" for the sake of convenience. They have done so not only through their television ads, but also through their packaging, using words like "natural," "whole grain," "real fruit," and "healthy." The only two things that are usually listed on the front of a package that I acknowledge as being trustworthy are the "USDA Organic" and/or "Certified Non-GMO Project" seals. In my humble opinion, these two have tremendous validity. Even so, there are deceptive "organic" labels. See the article on the Filtery website titled *What Does USDA Certified Organic Mean? Is it Really Healthier for You?* to learn more.[7]

The food industry has also used some deceptive tactics on their own websites. These tactics are possible in large part due to the millions (if not billions) of lobbying dollars funneled to our government every year, particularly to the Food and Drug Administration and the US Department of Agriculture, as well as Congress. This is not a "conspiracy theory;" it's the truth revealed by following the money spent annually on these efforts.

Many years ago, before I knew anything about which foods were healthy and which were not, I worked as an administrative assistant for the Milk & Ice Cream Association (now called the International Dairy Foods Association or IDFA). This is a lobbying organization, although at the time I truly did not know what that meant. I worked there for 5 years, and one of the things we did every year was host a huge ice cream party on Capitol Hill for all the Senators, Representatives, and their staff. Talk about getting to them through their stomachs! More accurately, it played to their addictions. This was a huge event, with hundreds of gallons of ice cream donated by all the dues-paying members of the Association.

One of the many responsibilities of the Association was to lobby Congress for food labeling protections. At the time, this Association

---

7 "Filtery" website entitled: *"What Does USDA Certified Organic Mean? Is it Really Healthier for You?"*

was on the same floor and right next door to the Sugar Association—imagine that—and one of our executives was on their board. Ooh, had I only known then what I know now—and as I look back on it, I recall having multiple doctor appointments in those five years for chronic headaches and digestive problems. Perhaps it had something to do with all the endless dairy and ice cream products I had free access to. Surely not.

In doing research for this book, I learned that a large conglomerate food company also owns a national weight loss company. While the parent company claims to care about health and nutrition, and manufactures "nutritional" supplements as well as pharmaceutical medications, their other products can lead to malnourishment and chronic illness. They also sell synthetic supplements and toxic drugs. I encourage you to do some research of your own on the companies whose foods you are consuming. I could write a whole book solely on food companies and their deceptions, but I want to keep my spirit, soul, and body as positive as possible, so I'll forgo that book for now!

One more tidbit of information about the big food industries and then I'll move on. The trade association for registered dietitians is the Academy of Nutrition and Dietetics (AND), and this organization lists Coca-Cola, PepsiCo, and Kellogg's among their corporate sponsors. I recall several years ago attending a continuing education seminar where the instructor shared a story with us. He was invited to be a speaker for one of their breakout sessions at their annual convention that year. He took some pictures while he was there—he was quite in awe, as were we. There were banners hanging in the convention hall of the various corporate sponsors and, in addition to the ones mentioned above and others, the Sugar Association was also present. Follow the money.

You might say "so what?" to all of this. Well, if you recall, packaged and processed foods (and sugars—which we will cover next) cause *inflammation* in the body, and inflammation is at the root of the chronic and degenerative diseases. These packaged/processed foods and sugars are also a huge culprit for children diagnosed with Attention Deficit Disorder (ADD) and Attention Deficit Hyperactivity Disorder (ADHD) and pose adverse effects to children with autism. The government entities that lead us to believe they are here to protect us and keep us safe and healthy are being bribed to turn a blind eye to the very things that are killing us.

In addition to sugar, there are many other toxic ingredients that are killers in these packaged and processed foods. Nitrates and nitrites, used as preservatives, are especially found in processed foods and are highly toxic. Aspartame and other artificial sweeteners are highly toxic to the nervous system. Next to cigarettes, consuming diet soda is probably the worst thing we can do to our bodies, and regular sodas run a close third. Monosodium glutamate (MSG) is also a highly toxic substance found in a tremendous amount of not only the packaged foods, but most of the foods in restaurants as well. I remember a chef who worked for a high-end restaurant telling me that even the restaurant he worked at used MSG to enhance the flavor of their foods. Food dyes of any color are found in so many foods, and these too, are very, very toxic. Other ingredients that we need to be aware of include wheat, corn, and soy (unless organic or non-GMO), and any word you cannot pronounce. This list really is a lot longer, and I encourage you to look up hidden ingredients in your foods—you will be shocked at what passes for "generally safe."

There are more than 3,000 hidden chemicals in our packaged foods these days, and they are very harmful to the body. These are ingredients that the body does not naturally produce or need to function. This is a tremendous burden to the body, particularly the liver.

Now there are some foods that come in a package that are reasonably safe to eat—but how do you know which are and which aren't? Start by ignoring what is printed on the front of the package (i.e., ignore the marketing ploy) and look at the back. Not the "Nutritional Facts" chart but the "Ingredients." This is the very first thing you should always read. The longer the list of ingredients and the more words you can't pronounce, the more processed, less nutritional, and more toxic it is and the more you should avoid it.

It used to be that the first ingredient listed was the dominant ingredient in the product. That is not necessarily true these days. Since light has been shed on the harm of sugars, the food companies now break down those various sugar sources and list them separately. They can do that because our government allows it. So even though sugar may, in total, be the largest quantity ingredient, it might not be listed first, even though sugar is sugar as far as the body is concerned.

When choosing the foods to eat, ask yourself two things: is this real food, and is this a food that heals or a food that kills? If I can go out into the field or the orchard and pick it off the tree or eat it out of the garden just as it is, provided it has not been genetically modified or sprayed with toxic chemicals, it's likely a food that heals. If it's in a package, with a list of ingredients a mile long that I can't pronounce, it's likely a food that kills.

I have already mentioned some of the symptoms and health conditions caused or exacerbated by packaged/processed foods. To recap, these are obesity, heart disease, thyroid problems, diabetes, osteoporosis, autoimmune diseases, ADD/ADHD, autism, insomnia, cancer, acid reflux, digestive disorders, kidney disease, gout, hormone imbalances, low libido, and much, much more. If you are struggling with *any* kind of symptom or health condition, please look at the foods you are eating.

Before you open your hand and your mouth to pop that drug in your body for the symptoms you are experiencing, remove the offending foods first—all fast food, fried food, packaged/processed foods and sugars. You will be *amazed* at just how good you might feel and just how healthy you can truly become!

The Truth about Sugar

As I've mentioned, I grew up in the 60s and 70s when the processed food and fast-food industries were *booming!* I remember childhood favorites like Tang, Kool-Aid, Pop tarts, Twinkies, Hostess Ho Ho's, Quisp & Quake Cereal, Cap'n Crunch, and many more as well as when that first McDonald's opened in my hometown. I am probably stirring up memories for some of you, too. There is one common denominator for all these products and companies—you got it—SUGAR!

Now, the sugar I'm talking about here isn't your grandma's or great-grandma's sugar—real natural sugars like honey, maple syrup, and even molasses. It's processed sugars, and even processed crackers, pasta, breads, etc., that turn to sugar.

There was a childhood obesity study done by the University of California, San Francisco (UCSF) a while back, and as part of their research they looked at the breads available in the grocery store. Thirty-four out of the 35 breads they researched had high fructose corn syrup in them. This ingredient is SUGAR!

NOTE: Some hidden (and toxic) names for sugar: high fructose corn syrup, corn syrup, dextrose, sucrose, and fructose.

In his book *Salt, Sugar, Fat,* Michael Moss revealed that some of the fast-food restaurants even put sugar in their salt, which they then use on their French fries and other products! Remember, these companies have leading scientists working to determine precisely just how much sugar or salt is the tipping point that will make you come back for more. They are literally and intentionally causing addictions in not only you, but also your children, to these food-like substances, which in turn is killing us. It is no wonder we have a society that is at least 50 percent overweight and 35 percent obese—and growing (no pun intended!). When the body has too much sugar that cannot get burned off, it turns to fat. But there is something even more ominous about sugar: cancers, chronic degenerative diseases, and even autoimmune diseases *thrive* on sugars, which have an acidic pH. Sugar is the fuel that keeps these diseases alive, thriving—and yes, growing—when in an acidic environment in our bodies.

Yet conventional medicine does not seem to embrace this. In fact, I have heard too many stories where people with active cancer in their bodies are told to eat literally anything they can and want, including sugars, just to keep the calories in them. My sister-in-law, who was receiving chemotherapy for breast cancer that had spread to her liver, was given donuts to eat every time she went in for her cancer treatment. Seriously, I struggle to make sense of this. Even if you didn't agree or know that cancers feed on sugar, it still is common knowledge that, at the very least, sugar does not have any nutritional benefit to the body. If someone is receiving chemotherapy for cancer, they are very, very sick; why would this be the practice with such a patient?

NOTE: 4 grams of sugar = roughly 1 teaspoon: think about this measurement every time you look at how much sugar is in a product (and you *should* look *every* time).

A common 20-ounce sports drink contains 32 grams of sugar—or about eight teaspoons—imagine that! Picture yourself serving up EIGHT TEASPOONS of sugar into your coffee for example! I think even those who like a little coffee with their sugar would say that is a lot. Another example is the single cup of low-fat yogurt that contains up to 47 grams of sugar, which is 12 teaspoons! But the deception here is in the way it is labeled on the package—in "grams" not "teaspoons"—something that is more relatable to most of us. For more information on sugar, see the article on the Alliance for Natural Health's website.[8] We will talk more about the adverse effects of sugar in Section 3.

Sugar Addiction—It's Real!

Sugar is also very addictive. It doesn't just trigger the body's addictive mechanism in the brain for *sugar*, but for *anything* that a person might have addictive tendencies toward, including alcohol, drugs, and food-like substances.

I worked at an addiction recovery center for women for a while, where the volunteers and even the staff just didn't get that this was not good for the ladies we served. They would bring cakes, cookies, and all kinds of other junk food in for the ladies because "they loved them!" Sadly, they did not recognize that their love was harming these ladies— possibly hindering their recovery more than even the ladies realized. We all have got to stop using toxic sugary foods to show love and reward.

8 https://anh-usa.org/would-you-put-eight-teaspoons-of-sugar-in-your-water/

An elementary school where I once volunteered gave the children ice cream bars as rewards for good grades. There was an actual ice cream cooler like you would see in a convenience store in the school cafeteria. These were the same children that they handed the ADD and ADHD medications to just hours before.

The same was true for the soup kitchen that was across the street. I have absolutely no doubt that every single marginalized person that walked through those doors was chronically ill. I remember one time being there and observing a lot of the folks drinking something bright blue—likely "blue dye # whatever" in those drinks. The food that was being served that day was white and lifeless—full of empty carbs and lacking any nutrients. When I asked the director why they couldn't serve something more nutritious, his reply was that they had to serve what was donated to them. Unfortunately, even our educated, financially stable, loving community of donors were serving from a place of not only ignorance but harm. We have a long way to go regarding educating people on the truth about wellness.

Here are some symptoms of sugar imbalances:

Symptoms of Hypoglycemia (low blood sugar):

- Having increased energy after meals
- Cravings for sweets between meals
- Irritability when meals are missed
- Dependency on coffee and sugar for energy
- Becoming lightheaded if meals are missed
- Eating to relieve fatigue
- Feeling shaky, jittery, or tremulous
- Feeling agitated and nervous

- Becoming easily upset
- Poor memory, forgetfulness
- Blurred vision

Symptoms of Insulin Resistance:

- Fatigue after meals
- General fatigue
- Constant hunger
- Craving for sweets or relieved by eating them
- Must have sweets after meals
- Waist girth equal to or larger than hip girth
- Frequent urination
- Increased appetite and thirst
- Difficulty losing weight
- Migrating aches and pains

Symptoms of Sugar Hangover:

- Fuzzy thinking or foggy mind
- Fatigue or sleepiness after meals
- Gas, bloating, or extended stomach after meals
- Headache
- Joint pain
- Constipation
- Diarrhea
- Skin problems
- Allergy symptoms

Emotional Symptoms of Sugar Hangover:

- Mood swings like emotional highs and then lows (anger, sadness, lack of willpower, depression, etc.)
- Feelings similar to having too much alcohol—and there's a reason for that

Physical Effects of Sugar Hangover:

- Kidneys are affected
- Liver is compromised
- Stomach issues
- Small intestines not functioning optimally
- Dehydration
- Electrolyte imbalances
- Gastrointestinal disturbances
- Sleep disruption

What about Meat?

I believe that God made animals for us to consume for our nourishment and health. If you are vegetarian or vegan or any other variation of these or believe otherwise and choose not to consume animal products, that's fine too. You must determine what works best for you and the health of your body. The most important point about eating any animal product is if you choose to do so, please be sure it is grass-fed, free-range, with no growth hormones or antibiotics injected into it and no GMO feed. It's *these* substances that are the culprit of animal products and that give animal foods a bad rap.

Livestock raised conventionally are routinely injected with growth hormones and antibiotics to grow the animals bigger, which also grows us bigger and indirectly gets those harmful antibiotics into our bodies—most of the time unknown to us. It's a huge harmful snowball effect.

When buying meat or eggs, look for Hormone-Free/ rB-GH-Free on the label. This label means that the farmer has chosen not to inject his or her cows or chickens with any artificial growth hormones (like rBGH, a genetically engineered growth hormone). The label is also used on other animal products where the animal was raised without growth hormones or steroids.

A Word of Caution

Folks who don't consume animal products, especially those who don't do so for their own ethical or spiritual reasons, seem to load up on carbs as the replacement food. Typically, it is the wrong kind of carbs—processed carbs for example, or carbs that have been genetically modified, sprayed with pesticides, high in gluten, etc. While we are on the subject, let's talk more about grains.

The Truth about Grains

I was a "carboholic" until I was in my early 40s. Pasta, bread, crackers—you name it, I loved them! I first became aware of this being a problem when I initially consulted a colleague to assess my health. She gave me a diet log form to keep track of all the food I ate and when I ate for an entire week.

I met with her the following week, and she took her big red pen and started circling all the "sugars" I was eating! I started to disagree. I truly was not a sugarholic, but I sure did love my "salty crunchy!" And that's what she was circling: Cheez-its for mid-morning snack, Cheez-its for mid-afternoon snack, Cheez-its for bedtime snack—

whoa! I was not only a "saltaholic" I was a "Cheez-itsaholic!" There are several problems here; those Cheez-its, and pretty much any other salty/crunchy snack food, are empty calories. There is no nutritional value whatsoever in these packaged and processed foods. While these types of foods may not be sweet, they still, however, turn to sugar, which eventually turns to fat if they are not quickly burned off. Now, I can already see the "wheels of workarounds" going through your heads! No, you cannot pop a handful of Cheez-its in your mouth and then go out and run a mile thinking you are home free! The body doesn't work that way. And that leads me to the third problem: these foods are not only devoid of any nutrients but also rob the body of the nutrients it does have. Our minerals like calcium (no, the "cheese" in Cheez-its is not real cheese any longer, and it is not fortified with calcium!), magnesium (the master mineral), potassium, and sodium (which we need in the right form).

Another deception is when processed food manufacturers put "made with whole grains" on the front of their packaging. What they aren't telling you is, while there might have been some whole grains in that batch of ingredients when it first started, the life of those grains was quickly killed off as soon as the processing took place.

But the biggest challenge with whole grains is that unless you are eating organic and non-GMO grains, you are consuming genetically modified grains, which are sprayed with cancer-causing chemicals to keep the pests and bugs off the plants and treated with toxic fertilizer. These same grains are not only sold to packaged/processed food manufacturers, but they are also sold to dairy and meat farmers as feed for their livestock. The cows, chickens, and pigs eat these toxic grains, and we indirectly consume these GMO products when we eat their meat and eggs.

The purpose of the producers genetically modifying these organisms is so they can produce more grain in an unnatural way and grow the livestock bigger and faster in unnatural ways, which in turn grows us bigger and faster in unnatural ways.

Another challenge with grains that are made into pastas, breads, sweets, and other baked goods is that they are the fuel for what is too common, especially for women, the candida yeast overgrowth.

So, if you are going to consume grains, be sure that they are organic and/or non-GMO.

Candida

Candida is a type of yeast that is found in the body. At an acceptable level, it can co-exist with us, but when its levels are too high, it can wreak havoc with our health. This is called candidiasis. Women are more prone to this than men, but men can be susceptible as well. Yeast feeds on sugars of all kinds, including natural healthy sugars like fruits. An overgrowth of yeast, vaginally as well as systematically throughout the whole body, causes a multitude of health problems. The symptoms are numerous, including skin, digestion, joints, even emotional and brain health problems.

When candida is too high, it also floods the body with a toxic by-product called acetaldehyde, which produces symptoms like an alcohol hangover. Acetaldehyde is poisonous to your tissues, is not easily eliminated, and accumulates in the brain, spinal cord, and muscles. Keeping in mind that your heart and intestines are muscles, you may now understand why you have symptoms of brain fog, muscle weakness, and even digestive pain. Unfortunately, as we just talked about, the typical processed foods and drinks on the market have so much hidden sugar that the average American is (often unknowingly) consuming approximately one-half cup of sugar per day.

This is just one serious example of the consequences and adverse impacts on our health from consuming processed sugars. Do yourself and your family a huge favor and eliminate all processed sugars from your diet and your life. If you don't do anything else after reading this book, do this. I promise you it will make a huge difference for you wholistically—mentally, emotionally, physically, and even spiritually.

Noninflammatory Foods

Let's next consider the foods that heal, the noninflammatory foods. These foods are healthy and healing to the body. You can have 4,000 calories of vegetables if you want, and you will not get fat. And truthfully, the same goes for the good fats—well okay, maybe not 4,000 calories of coconut oil, but these good fats will not "make you fat!" Here is the short-list of non-inflammatory foods:

- Fruits
- Vegetables
- Nuts & Seeds
- Good Fats (e.g., avocados, flax seed, olive oil, coconut oil—LOVE my coconut oil!)
- Water

There are many wonderful recipes out there using the short list of noninflammatory foods. Look up "raw food" recipes or "alkalizing foods" or even noninflammatory food recipes. You will be amazed at what you can do with fruits, vegetables, nuts, seeds, and good fats. And they truly are delicious! So, before you say "this takes too much time" or "I can't afford to eat real food"—remember the mental quadrant of the health pie (time management, budget, etc.) can have a tremendous impact on our health. I encourage you, if you find yourself making these statements, to reprioritize your time and/or your budget. It literally can mean life or death to you. For now, I am just asking you to trust me and give this new paradigm a try.

The Truth about Fruits and Vegetables

Growing up, most vegetables I ate came from a can. We might have a so-called "salad" with maybe two or three different vegetables in it, several times a week. I remember absolutely *hating* green peas; they came from a can, and they were so mushy! It wasn't until I started waitressing as a young adult at a high-end restaurant where they served fresh vegetables that I started loving them—what a delight! Thankfully, I absolutely *love* fresh peas today.

I think vegetables are the ultimate food. We should consume as much of them as we possibly can: fresh first, then frozen, and canned only as a last resort. Ideally, they would be organic no matter what form they are in. In fact, in a perfect world, the most nutritious meal would be raw, organic, local, and seasonal. Now I know this isn't always possible, even if you took the money factor out of it. In fact, not being able to afford fresh organic produce is the weakest excuse for not eating this way. Availability is usually more of a challenge for those living in smaller communities where the larger health food stores like Whole Foods, Trader Joe's, etc., are not readily available.

In all of my schooling and studying—post-doctorate classes, continuing-ed seminars, books on natural health and healing, conversations with colleagues—the number of *calories* an individual should consume on any given day is *never* part of the healing protocol. Yes, calories are important—they are fuel but that should not be our primary measuring stick as to the foods we choose. *Nutrients* should always be the priority. You can eat 500 calories of ice cream daily and lose weight but obviously as your only food source it would be unhealthy and lack nutrients. Or you can eat 4,000 calories of vegetables and achieve both: lose weight *and* receive amazing nutrients. I promise you, if all you could afford was money for vegetables and nothing else, you would not starve to death. It would take quite a while before your body starts lacking other vital nutrients like proteins and fats, which are vital in the right form as well. If your dollars only provide vegetables, then so be it, at least for the time being. You just might heal your body of the chronic degenerative diseases that are keeping you from working a better paying job or even working at all. Then you can afford to buy some protein and good fats.

Fruits are a similar story. However, I do raise caution, especially for women, that if you are struggling with candidiasis (candida yeast overgrowth), then you will need to totally avoid all sugars, including fruits, until that is cleared up. Since yeast feeds on sugars, this will take tremendous diligence to avoid *all* sugars, as any little bit keeps that yeast thriving and growing.

That is one challenge I have with the keto diet, which prohibits all fruits except some berries. There are some nutrients that can only be obtained from real fruit; avoiding fruits is to deprive the body of these vital nutrients. The bottom line is God made all real food for the nourishment of our bodies, including fruits.

The Truth about Nuts and Seeds

If you are 50 years old or older, you might be familiar with Euell Gibbons, the tree-hugger from California who only ate nuts and berries—or at least that's the image I have of him! He was a fad in the 60s from the hippie generation eating wheat bran and other cereals that tasted and felt like gravel in your mouth. Consequently, this might turn you off when you hear "eat nuts and seeds."

One year, as my health journey continued to progress (and it still is!), I committed to eating nothing but organic foods. My first trip to the grocery store was sticker shock to say the least! I will not argue that organic food is more expensive than eating genetically modified food-like substances. I was also in for a culture shock. It took some time getting adjusted to the truth of real food, and humility to admit that I had not been eating real food for a long time. Even worse, I realized some of the health challenges I had experienced in the past were of my own ignorant food and lifestyle choices (remember all that dairy and ice cream I consumed?!) not to mention my financial priorities.

The foods that weren't really on my radar up to this point were nuts and seeds. These are not cheap. In fact, I still get the conventionally grown walnuts and cashews; the organic price remains out of my budget, no matter how high of a priority healthy eating is for me.

A few years later, when I committed to eating an all-raw food diet, the cost of groceries was somewhat higher when I began exchanging organic meats on the grocery list for a large variety of nuts and seeds.

In fact, the healthiest I ever felt was the year I committed to eating an all-raw food diet. Now you might be asking yourself "did she eat raw meat?" No, that is not what I mean by a raw food diet. Nor is it simply just eating straight up vegetables, fruits, nuts, and seeds in their basic form. You might be surprised to know that there is a whole other world of food preparation and dining out there beyond our standard American diet. I found it a truly exciting way to prepare food, and again I felt amazing! I lost 25 of the 30 pounds I gained during menopause, I had tremendous energy, slept great, my digestive health was beautiful—it was amazing! Unfortunately, I started dating a fella who still preferred to eat the (old) government food-pyramid way that he adopted in his military days. I served him some raw veggie burgers early on in our dating and to his credit, he was straight up honest; after a few bites he pushed it away and said, "I can't eat this!" From then on, I compromised a bit when we went out to eat; I ordered the healthiest choice on the menu and when I prepared a meal for us, I would do the same. When I was preparing meals for myself, I continued with my raw food dishes. You might have to do the same. All I can say is, I am at my best when I am eating real food, and ideally raw.

Nuts and seeds are a strong base for most of these dishes, especially the desserts. Yes, I said desserts! Maybe that will be a great way to dip your toes in the raw food diet: start with desserts.

Of course, nuts and seeds have tremendous nutritional value. They are a great source of healthy fats that our bodies need (and we will talk about next), as well as a great source of protein and fiber too. They are also high in vitamin E and magnesium—and they are noninflammatory!

The Truth about Fat

Do you remember the "fat free" diet craze of the 1990s? I do; there was some kind of cookie that touted "fat free" that everyone was buying off the shelves. Nonfat milk, nonfat ice cream and so much more. This led people to believe "a diet high in fat = a fat body." Then the craze moved onto sugar-free diets, and now it's carb-free diets. Prior to the 1990s, it was low-calorie diets. I wonder what it will be 10 years from now.

Of course, to go along with all these food crazes came the diets themselves. I can remember eating a very low-calorie diet shortly out of high school. And honestly, when I look back at pictures of myself even 20 years out of high school, I was thin—skinny was more like it. Middle school pictures? I looked like mom didn't feed me much! That low-calorie diet generally consisted of cottage cheese, tomato, and one hard-boiled egg. Remember when bagels were the health craze? I guess because that's what Hollywood was doing, it was the "diet of beauties!" Not sure why anyone would think a flavorless, heavier-than-lead piece of baked bleached flour could be "healthy"—especially when it was slathered with cream cheese. These are the types of things we bought into.

Then there were, and still are, several weight loss companies. As women started working outside the home more, these diet programs then also produced frozen meals and "shakes." What these meals do, and any of these diets for that matter, is simply control your calorie intake and make someone else rich.

My same friend who wouldn't eat my raw veggie burgers cuts every single bit of fat off any meat or fish he might be consuming—he is *that* obsessed about not eating fat. Now, to his credit, he barely has a stitch of fat on his body, but I think it has more to do with the fact that he is an Army Ranger, and he is 100 percent committed to their creed "keep your body fit." I also believe it has to do with exercising and, being a bachelor who doesn't really cook, his calorie intake is probably low as well. I don't believe it has much, if anything, to do with not consuming fat, although he is probably consuming more fat than he realizes—he is a pretty big dairy eater, milk and cheese in particular.

The point I want to drive home is that our bodies need *good* fats. Our brains need good fats as do our cell walls. Eating fat in our diets does not make us fat.

Good Fats versus Bad

The truth is there are good fats and there are bad fats. The trans fats and hydrogenated fats are quite inflammatory, and yes, you do want to stay away from those as much as possible. Good fats like polyunsaturated and monounsaturated fats are necessary for our health. All our cell walls are made up of fat—whether good or bad, you make that choice—but the fact remains they are made up of fats. Would you want flimsy, poor quality "walls" in your house (your body) or would you want sound, solid walls—the kind that the big bad wolf couldn't blow down?

Our immune system requires fats. Our brain is made up of 60 percent fat. Our organs are protected by fat. You decide the quality by the kind of fats you feed your body.

Good fat is very, very vital to the health of our bodies. Some examples of good fats include flax seed and other nuts and seeds, olive oil, avocados, and coconut oil just to name a few. I love anything coconut, especially because it has so many healing properties.

Our taste buds have been sabotaged into craving the wrong kinds of fats (like salty crunchy processed foods), and some of us even started on solid foods with bad fats when we were babies.

I recall vacationing in Aruba with a couple of high school classmates to celebrate our 60th birthdays. There was a man with a coconut truck on one end of the island selling real coconut water and demonstrating how to open it up the right way—yes, there is a true art to doing this! I was so excited to drink some fresh coconut water, so I bought some. My friends asked for a taste, and one of them made a face and said, "That doesn't even *taste* like coconut!" She just saw the man pour it right from the real coconut but was deceived into believing that something she had from the grocery store (or worse, a pina colada somewhere!) was the real thing.

> *An article from the* Journal of American College of Nutrition *states that during the past several decades, reduction in fat intake has been the main focus of national dietary recommendations to decrease risk of coronary heart disease (CHD). Several lines of evidence, however, have indicated that types of fat have a more important role in determining risk of CHD than total amount of fat in the diet. Metabolic studies have long established that the type of fat, but not the total amount of fat, predicts serum cholesterol levels. In addition, results from epidemiologic studies and controlled clinical trials have indicated that replacing saturated fat with unsaturated fat is more effective in lowering risk of CHD than simply reducing total fat consumption. Moreover, prospective cohort studies and secondary prevention trials have provided strong evidence that an increasing intake of n-3 fatty acids from fish or plant sources substantially lowers the risk of cardiovascular mortality.*[9]

Remember, good fats are one of the noninflammatory foods, and our bodies need good fats. If you want to lose weight, or not gain it to begin with, consume a healthy balance of good fats.

---

9 (3)Types of dietary fat and risk of coronary heart disease: a critical review F B Hu et al J Am Coll Nutr. 2001 Feb;20(1):5-19.doi: 10.1080/07315724.2001.10719008

Definition of Fats according to the Harvard School of Public Health

Trans Fats are made by heating liquid vegetable oils in the presence of hydrogen gas and a catalyst, a process called hydrogenation. Partially hydrogenating vegetable oils makes them more stable and less likely to become rancid. This process also converts the oil into a solid, which makes them function as margarine or shortening.

Trans Fats are the worst type of fat for the heart, blood vessels, and rest of the body because they:

- Raise bad LDL and lower good HDL blood cholesterol
- Create inflammation
- Contribute to insulin resistance

Saturated Fats are mainly found in animal foods, but a few plant foods are also high in saturated fats, such as coconut, coconut oil, palm oil, and palm kernel oil.

Unsaturated Fats are predominantly found in foods from plants, such as vegetable oils, nuts, and seeds:

- Polyunsaturated Fats are found in high concentrations in sunflower, corn, soybean, and flaxseed oils, walnuts, flax seeds, and fish
- Omega-3 Fats are an important type of polyunsaturated fat. The body can't make these, so they must come from food.
- Monounsaturated Fats are found in high concentrations in olive, peanut, and canola oils; avocados; nuts such as almonds, hazelnuts, and pecans; and seeds such as pumpkin and sesame seeds.

The Truth About Water

Of course we already talked about water, but I put this on the list because pretty much any of our other liquid choices contrary to this are probably packaged, processed and/or high in sugar. Some herbal teas are healthy—but again, check your sources and labels on these—are they organic? Do they call themselves a "tea" but have other toxic ingredients added to them–like sugar, colorings, additives etc.? Coffee is fine in moderation, and the time of day it is consumed, and ideally organic. Is it disturbing your sleep, making you jittery? Are you dependent on it for energy? If so, look for the root cause of the lack of energy, you are not deficient in caffeine. And it is acidic, so again, moderation.

So, this is the short list of noninflammatory foods. This is an absolutely great place to make dietary changes. For starters, I would suggest choosing one category from the inflammatory foods list and totally eliminate it. If you already don't eat much fast food, then start there if you must—for a week. Check it off your goals list as a win, and move onto the next least invasive food-like substance you consume. Eliminate it for a period of time, and keep working your way off the inflammatory foods list. You will start finding yourself wanting and probably even needing more food and calories to consume. Don't replace one bad item with another, but instead add a noninflammatory food in its place. Start exchanging the bad for the good; the inflammatory for the noninflammatory.

Call to Action: Change of any kind is a process. To borrow a saying from Alcoholics Anonymous (AA) , take it "one day at a time." Just keep taking the next best step forward every day. Stretching yourself a little more—eliminating the foods that kill from your diet, and adding the healthy, life-giving nutrients in. Don't stop just because you've lost weight, or even because a chronic health condition has been cleared up—and in time, you will lose weight, and you will become healthier. Remember the "Wellness is Not" and the "Wellness Is" truths from chapters 2 and 3: Wellness is not easy, but it does take a commitment, and it is a lifestyle change. I believe when you start making these changes to your diet and your life, you *will* see positive change, it's a beautiful thing, and it's empowering. Look forward to it!

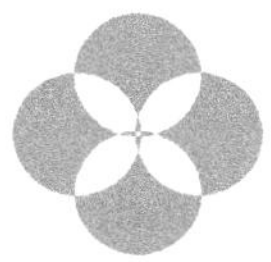

SECTION 2

A Little Anatomy Can Go a Long Way

I'm a why person–and maybe even a little arrogant at times. If someone gives me instructions to do something and I understand why I am supposed to be doing it a specific or certain way, I will be much more compliant. But if I don't have clarity on the "why", I have a tendency to think I know a better way than the person who gave me the instructions. Especially if someone tells me I "can't" do something–oh, my defiance kicks in and I think "I'll show you!" For example, years ago, I was told not to eat junk food because it was not good for me. My mind interpreted that to mean that it would put weight on me. Well, I didn't have a weight problem so I didn't heed that wise advice. If I had known it was because it caused inflammation in my body and I was experiencing joint pain, that would have been a different story—I would have complied right away. Have you been there?

I also learned as I started down the path of the functional medicine world, that I truly didn't appreciate how all the various parts of the body worked together as a whole—and how they could influence each other. I was also beginning to appreciate the "root cause and effect" philosophy, and that certain organs or systems in the body played huge roles where the roots quite often lied.

This section will help you understand the basic roles and functions of these major organs and systems. Once you have this valuable understanding, it will make a whole lot more sense as you work toward healing your body.

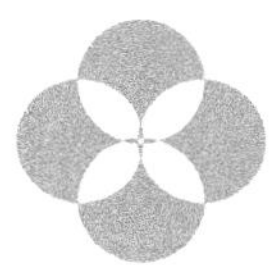

CHAPTER 7

Four Organs and Systems of the Body That Can Extend Your Health!

"For just as in one [physical] body we have many parts, and these parts do not all have the same function or special use, so we, who are many, are [nevertheless just] one body in Christ, and individually [we are] parts one of another [mutually dependent on each other]."

—Romans 12:4-5 AMP

When I was in chiropractic school, I learned a whole lot more than just the bones in our back. In fact, most people are surprised to learn that chiropractors spend the same number of hours in the classroom for their doctorate as a medical doctor. The main difference is that medical doctors study pharmacology in great detail, while chiropractors get very little of this topic. On the flip side, chiropractors study in great detail about nutrition, whereas medical docs study this minimally, if at all.

The study of anatomy is just as rigorous in chiropractic school as it is in medical school. This is because chiropractors are concerned with the function of the whole body. One of the things we did was dissect cadavers for three semesters. It was really fascinating. I share all of this to simply put emphasis on the depth of studying we had to do to understand the human body, including the adrenal glands. We didn't just learn where they are, but the physiology and function of them.

Fast forward three or four years, and I am now being doctored by a fellow chiropractor, who is practicing functional medicine. In fact, it was her care of me that inspired me to take my chiropractic career to the next level. When she started talking about the adrenal glands and how mine were out of balance, though, I had no choice but to pretend I knew fully what she was talking about! But behind the scenes in the archives of my brain I was trying to not only remember what they were and where they were, but what in the heck did they do?!

I say all of this because I don't want you to feel embarrassed or ignorant for not knowing much—if anything—about most of your body parts, let alone how they function. You're not alone, most people don't understand their own body processes very well. But fear not, a quick anatomy overview is in store for you next!

I'd like to bring your attention to four often-overlooked organs and systems, and how they can be the root of many of the chronic degenerative diseases experienced today. They are the adrenal glands, the liver, the digestive system, and the brain. We'll go into more detail with each of them next. Please note that this is not an in-depth anatomy lesson, so I encourage you to explore more on your own as your curiosity prompts you to learn how each of these vital organs and/or systems functions. I will also introduce you to an area that too often seems to be overlooked regarding having an adverse effect on our health and that is trauma—especially childhood trauma, and one of the primary results of that trauma leading to addiction. And trauma is stress.

We'll begin with the adrenal glands which release a hormone called cortisol to respond to all stress and inflammation in the body.

The Truth about the Adrenal Glands

The adrenal glands are two triangular-shaped glands that sit on top of each kidney. These two little glands have so many *major* functions, and yet unless there is a full-blown pathological problem with them (which is fairly uncommon, thankfully), they are tremendously overlooked by traditional medicine. Yet, these tiny glands are so vital to our life and our health that we can't live without at least one of them.

Let's first cover the different functions of the adrenal glands, and then we'll go into more detail about the good and bad effects they have on our health.

Cortisol—What is It?

The first major role of the adrenal glands is to release a hormone called cortisol. Too little of this hormone makes us vulnerable to inflammation and hypoglycemia. Too much makes us vulnerable to autoimmune diseases, high blood pressure, type 2 diabetes, and a lowered immunity which makes us susceptible to viruses, bacteria, and cancer.

There are four words that are interchangeable: stress, inflammation, acidic pH, and toxic. If you don't remember anything else from this book, remember this statement. I repeat, there are four words that are interchangeable: stress, inflammation, acidic pH, and toxic.

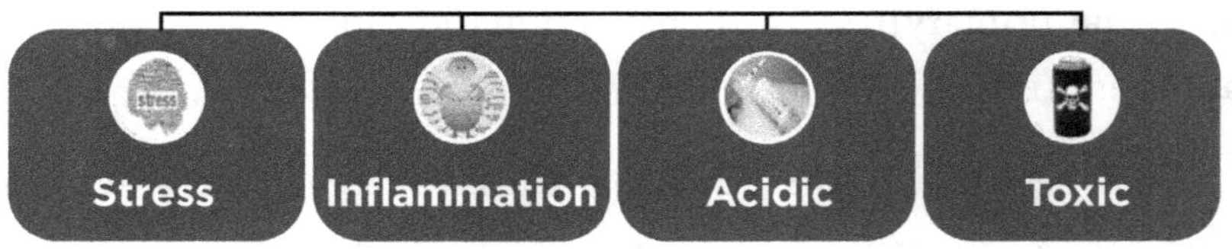

Typically, the first thing we think of when we hear the word "stress" is mental and/or emotional stress, such as family, financial, health, or career issues. But stress is also physical (e.g., having surgery, breaking your arm, or over-exercising). There are chemical stresses as well, like the foods we eat, the air we breathe, the water we drink, medications, etc. Some things are more in our control than others in regard to minimizing the stresses to the adrenal glands; our diet is one of them. Cigarettes and sodas of any kind are probably the two worst chemical assaults we make on our bodies.

Cortisol responds to all of these stressors. In time, this overworks the adrenal glands and throws them out of balance, which then affects all the other roles they perform as well.

Adrenal glands also release hormones called epinephrine and norepinephrine. These are your "fight or flight" hormones. If a bear is chasing you in the woods, these hormones tell the digestive system, urinary system, and other functions to slow down while at the same time kicking the muscles, heart, and lungs into high gear: You need to run, not digest your food—a bear is chasing you!! This is that "adrenaline rush" we all probably have experienced at some time in our lives—maybe not due to a bear, but perhaps a quick scare of some other kind. Helping us with these things is partly why we have adrenal glands.

However, when we are constantly on the go, foot on the gas pedal of life full throttle, 24/7 for days, weeks, months, and years on end, we can burn out our adrenal glands. Once that happens, they are not able to properly perform their functions, leading to a multitude of health problems. You may have possibly heard people refer to their overworked adrenals, and wondered what that is. Well, now you know.

Epinephrine and norepinephrine are brain chemicals too, and they work with our other brain chemicals such as dopamine, serotonin, GABA, leptin, and melatonin. As we learned, these hormones regulate our mood, appetite, sleep, and so much more. If the adrenals are out of balance because these hormones are constantly being released, we could experience symptoms like anxiety, depression, insomnia, etc.

Another role of the adrenal glands is to tell the liver to release glucose, our body's natural energy source and our brain's fuel. Glucose is vital to life and we cannot live without it. This is why we can't live without at least one adrenal gland. Symptoms like brain fog, lack of energy/fatigue, and blood sugar highs and lows can be a result of the adrenals being out of balance. And of course chronic diseases like diabetes and insulin-resistance can be traced back to the adrenals being out of balance as well.

Cortisol is also upstream of the hormonal pathways that are constantly flowing in the body. In particular and in part, it is formed from cholesterol and then ultimately plays a role in the production of our reproductive hormones like estrogen, progesterone, and testosterone.

Lastly, the adrenals release a hormone called aldosterone that signals the kidneys to regulate the fluid levels in our body, particularly those at work inside and outside our cells, including the blood cells. Things like edema and blood pressure imbalances can be a result of the adrenals being out of balance.

I also believe that stress and inflammation are huge culprits and essentially the "root" of not only the adrenal glands being thrown out of balance, but the root of all chronic and degenerative diseases.

I hope you can already see how important the adrenal glands are to not only some major functions of our body, but to our overall health. Later we'll discuss some specific health conditions that can be a result of the adrenals being out of balance, and how you can reverse these and restore the body back to good health. For now, I just want you to have a basic understanding of where these glands are and some of their major functions.

Think about your own life. I would like to suggest that you make a list of some of the stressors in your own life—mental/emotional, chemical, and physical—and make a plan for changing these. Here's a tip: The chemical stresses are usually easier to eliminate than the mental/emotional ones, so start there. Other stressors are:

- Lack of deep sleep—going to bed too late, and/or waking in the middle of the night and not being able to go back to sleep, are some examples.
- Eating an inflammatory diet—fast food, fried food, *packaged and processed foods*, and sugars (this one is huge). The foods that heal or are noninflammatory are fruits, vegetables, nuts and seeds, good fats, and water.

- Being dehydrated—water flushes the waste and toxins out of the body on a daily basis. If you are dehydrated, these toxins stay in you causing inflammation in the body.
- Lack of exercise—prayer and exercise are much better stress relievers than an anxiety or depression medication.
- Nerve interference in the spine—the nerve roots coming from the thoracic spine (the middle/lower part of your back) go to the adrenal glands. Most people have nerve interference unless they are having their spines maintained with the help of a chiropractor.
- Dietary and lifestyle choices that directly affect your health—cigarettes and sodas can lead to a decline in your health, as do gluten, cow's milk (including ice cream, even when it's organic) and sugar. If you avoid these, you may very well see a tremendous improvement in your health from the inflammation they can cause. In fact, cow's milk is the number one hidden food sensitivity and very inflammatory (more about this in chapter 9). When we consume foods that we are knowingly or unknowingly sensitive to, they also can cause inflammation in the body. Avoiding hidden food sensitivities is very important for your children too—especially if they are struggling with attention problems, sleep problems, and/or autism.
- I mentioned lack of sleep as an example of physical stress to the body. As stated before, we need at least seven to nine hours of sleep per night. Here's why: The body can only repair and regenerate itself while we sleep, specifically between 10:00 p.m. and midnight. If you are not asleep by 10 p.m., you are short-changing your body's vital regeneration process.

When the body is stressed, certain nutrients are not absorbed by the body.

Here are some of the nutrients that are compromised when the body is stressed:

- Cholesterol
- Vitamins and minerals (e.g., B vitamins, magnesium, etc.)
- Enzymes
- Essential fatty acids
- Proteins
- Oxygen
- Glucose

There are also physical health problems that can occur as a direct result of the body being stressed. Here are a few:

- Anxiety
- Depression
- Digestive disorders
- Diabetes
- Hypoglycemia
- Hypertension
- Autoimmune disorders
- Cancer
- Obesity
- Arthritis

Stress: The Silent Killer

Let's delve in a little more about chemical stresses. If you do not benefit from anything else out of this book, please understand this: The foods you eat can either *kill* you or they can *heal* you.

I once had a conversation with a woman who ate a horrible diet; she had one child in the hospital with cancer, another who was autistic, and she herself was very unhealthy. Yet she was in total denial that her food choices had anything at all to do with her or her children's health problems. I promise you—they do! Please, please understand that fast foods, fried foods, *packaged and processed* foods, and sugars are *killing you and your family—quickly!*

Over the years, I've had multiple conversations with people who say their kids won't eat the good foods they try to feed them, so they have to buy the "junk" food. My response is "No, no, you do not!" Please realize when you compromise like this, whether for yourself or your children, you are literally feeding your family poison. You are not doing them a favor by feeding them chemical-laden food-like substances with *no nutritional value.* As the doctor used to tell my mom when she would complain that my one brother was a picky eater, "he will eat (the healthy foods) when he is hungry enough." Your child will not starve to death, contrary to what you might think.

I realize that it's not easy to make a quick change to your family's diet. So don't do it quickly. Begin to substitute healthier foods for the processed ones, and don't be surprised when your children don't want to eat it. It takes time to switch the palate from the junky food to the healthy foods. Remain steadfast. Be creative. But make the change.

It's not about how *full* or how satisfied one is; it's about how *nourished* one is. You are the parent, and it is *your* hard-earned money that is used to buy the groceries or pay the medical bills when they get sick—not to mention how your heart aches when they are feeling helpless. *You* should be telling *them* what to eat, not the other way around. You are the parent, and they are the children. Okay, so now I'm digressing, and I will step down from my soapbox (once again!). Back to the adrenals…

When you feed your body foods that are inflammatory, have an acidic pH, and/or are toxic, the created stress causes the adrenal glands to release cortisol. If this goes on long enough, the adrenal glands start "burning out," also affecting glucose levels, fluid levels, some brain chemical activity, and the reproductive hormones. Overworked adrenal glands can lead to a cascade of other health problems. These include blood sugar imbalances, high or low blood pressure, hormone imbalances, fatigue, irritability, depression, anxiety, insomnia, hot flashes, mood swings, low libido, low energy, slow metabolism, chronic fatigue, brain fog, and much more. The cortisol, in a sense, works closely with the immune system. If the adrenal glands are overworked and can't produce enough cortisol, the inflammation remains, and the immune system is lowered. More doors of disease are now opened like reduced immunity in general and cancers more specifically. This becomes a vicious cycle.

The immune system is the body's defense team. Think of it as your body's army and it only has a finite number of "soldiers." Cortisol makes up some of those "soldiers." When we eat an inflammatory diet, these "soldiers" are called upon unnecessarily, redirecting them from the more important battles they have to fight. There is only so much to go around; minimizing the stressors to our bodies that are within our control will support and enable our immune system, and support our body's army to function efficiently. Eliminating the most toxic and inflammatory substances (e.g., cigarette smoke, sodas, artificial sweeteners, fast food, fried food, processed and packaged foods, and sugars) will help put you on the fast-track to restoring good health to your body.

When you eat healing, noninflammatory foods, you are actually *building up* your "reserves." You are *boosting* your immune system and relieving your body of stress. Therefore, the cortisol does not have to be released nearly as much, allowing the adrenal glands to be replenished. In turn, they can do all their other tasks, such as release the proper amount of glucose, balance blood pressure, give energy, brain fuel, and stamina, and give the body the protection it needs against all the other stresses that are not within our control.

Whenever possible, eat fresh, uncooked vegetables, fruits, nuts and seeds, good fats, and water. These foods truly are HEALING! An endless number of recipes available on the internet these days will show you how to prepare these foods in tasty ways you would never have imagined; just search for "raw food recipes" and you will be amazed at what you can find.

Start thinking outside the box when it comes to new foods to eat, take control of your health, be empowered, be free. And know your health IS in your control!

The Truth About the Liver

The liver has over 500 functions that we know about; there are likely even more. I'll cover some of the main functions here. The liver synthesizes bile salts, which play a key role in fat digestion and the absorption of fat-soluble vitamins. Bile secretion is the main digestive function of the liver. Through the synthesis of plasma proteins, the liver maintains blood volume and controls blood coagulation. It also stores glucose, fat-soluble vitamins (A, D, E, K), and vitamin B12.

The liver also cleans the body of its toxins in a process called detoxification, and gets rid of bilirubin, cholesterol, and drugs through excretion. It is responsible for metabolizing carbohydrates, proteins, and fats, and also regulates blood glucose. The liver chemically alters or excretes thyroid hormones and steroid hormones. It activates Vitamin D and stores iron and copper, and removes cellular garbage, bacteria, and other substances through a process called "phagocytosis." It really is an amazing organ.

Whew! If I were the liver, I'd be tired by now from all that work! And yet this is just the tip of the iceberg of what all it is entrusted to do.

So How Does the Liver Get "Dirty?"

The processed foods we eat, the air we breathe, and the water we drink all affect the liver. Stress will also cause the body and the liver to be toxic. If the pH of the internal environment of our bodies is too acidic, the body is toxic. Just the natural process of cells dying off creates a waste product that the liver disposes of, and this is a lot of work. Mental/emotional stresses our bodies have been under, whether in the past year or the past 10 years, can also affect the liver. A major illness, surgery, loss of a loved one, loss of a job or home, relocation, marriage, divorce, childbirth—all kinds of major life events, good or bad, can cause stress to the body.

Some of the more common signs and symptoms of toxic buildup are allergies, arthritis, blood sugar problems, brain fog, carpal tunnel syndrome, chronic backache, chronic fatigue, colitis, constipation, headaches, hormonal problems, hot flashes, immune weakness, indigestion, gas, bloating, joint or muscle pain, mood changes, PMS, sinus congestion, skin conditions, and much more; the symptoms seem endless.

Why Do a Liver Detox?

Having said all of this, I encourage you to consider detoxifying your liver. The liver works exceptionally hard. I personally do a liver detox once a year and have been doing this for almost 20 years now. I usually do it at the beginning of the year, after the holidays have passed and as the new year begins.

For a long time, up until the past few years, I was doing the detox combined with a spiritual fast with the intent of giving the Lord my first of everything for the year. I figure if there is any organ or system of my body that is compromised, it would probably be my liver because of the 20+ years of heavy drinking I did. But 2022 was an extremely toxic year for me. Until that year, I think I took one prescription medication—an antibiotic for an abscessed tooth—in about 25 years. Then what? COVID-19. Probably like most of you, I was hit with COVID in January 2022, and it was all downhill from there that year. Until 2022, I truly had not been sick with anything other than an annual cold (and most of the time I wasn't sure that I even had that).

You may recall that in April 2022 I ended up with a kidney stone. It started with horrendous mid-back pain, so I went to my chiropractor twice. As it turned out, two days later, I started with right lower quadrant abdominal pain that would not relieve. I went to a primary care doctor who ordered a CT scan; lo and behold, there was the 9mm kidney stone. Several days later I went in to have it removed; after enduring the anesthesia, I woke up in what felt like a minute later (it was 45 minutes actually) for the doctor to tell me that there was no kidney stone when he went in—what?! Apparently, I had passed it over those couple days and never even knew it—thank you, Jesus! Although I was grateful, the downside was

I was given a very toxic anesthesia cocktail, including some fentanyl, for nothing. With toxins in my body, and the delay in completing my liver detox at the beginning of the year because of my having COVID, I did one following the kidney stone incident.

Then, later that year, I lost my job which caused mental and emotional stress, and was put under anesthesia for a *second* time to remove a teratoma tumor that was around my ovary. This was discovered in the results of the CT scan I had for the kidney stone. Whew! I don't know how people who are unhealthy and chronically ill for years do it.

I view every year as a new year and an opportunity to continue to take charge of my health. Thankfully I have been, or I have no doubt each of these scenarios could have been far worse. I share this story to convey that we can get hit with so many toxins throughout each year, and at least in my opinion, a liver detox is a must for me.

How To Do a Liver Detox

The protocol I used to put my patients on is very easy to do and not overly inconvenient. It's a 15-day program, you drink two essentially tasteless detox drinks a day, eat lean proteins and vegetables (ideally organic), take some prescribed supplements, and drink tons of clean water. The detox drinks make the toxins in the liver water soluble, and the toxins are then passed through the kidneys and out of the body through the urine. It's so easy and yet so important to do. The product I suggest is a professional-grade nutraceutical detox made by Biotics Research Corporation. To use this product for a liver detox, I would highly recommend either ordering through my professional link at: https://us.fullscript.com/welcome/jmckool or finding a wholistic practitioner who can order this for you. A listing is included at the end of this book in the Resources section.

If the Biotics product is out of your comfort area cost wise, my second best recommendation would be the 30-day Liver Detox by Renew Life: https://www.betteryourhealth.com/renewlife/product/liver-detox.

Even though Biotics' product can be fairly pricey, the effectiveness and quality of their detox makes it the right choice for me.

The Truth about the Digestive System

In reclaiming your health, another important aspect to address is bringing your digestive system back into balance.

Our body's digestion actually starts before food ever even enters our mouths. Think about biting into a bright, juicy, yellow lemon wedge—did your mouth just produce excess saliva? Mine did! The thought of food, the smell of food, even the sound of food cooking starts the digestive process going. Next, our stomach starts breaking that food down, getting it ready for the small intestines to pull out all of the delicious nutrients to feed and build our cells. Seventy percent of your immune system resides in the digestive system. The majority of the body's serotonin (the "feel good" hormone) is in the digestive system as well. The digestive system is where all the body's vitamins and minerals are reabsorbed and sent off to all the other parts of the body where they are utilized. And of course, without our large intestine, a lot of the body's waste would not be eliminated—thank God for this natural "garbage can" He built in us.

So, what makes up the digestive system? The main organs are the stomach, small intestine, and large intestine (also known as the colon). Other organs that contribute greatly to the digestive process are the gallbladder, liver, and pancreas. Believe it or not, the appendix has a role as well. When any one of these organs, in part or as a whole, are surgically removed, the body and the digestive system, in particular, are forever compromised. So please, consider and seek out ALL of your less invasive options *first* before having body parts removed. God put them there for a reason.

The Stomach

Once the teeth have broken down the food small enough to pass through your esophagus, it is then sent down to the stomach, where the first major step of the digestive process takes place. If the body is functioning optimally, hydrochloric acid (HCl) gets released to break the food down even further. This stomach acid is vital to the body for breaking down the foods before it can be passed on to the small intestines. But if there isn't enough stomach acid, the foods are only partially digested. At times when food is only partially digested, it comes back up through the esophagus bringing a little bit of stomach acid with it. This is known as acid reflux, which causes heartburn and possibly, over time, erosion of the esophagus.

The main means for the medical profession to diagnose the need for an antacid is simply based on the symptoms of acid reflux and heartburn. However, the symptoms for not enough stomach acid and too much are basically the same. More people don't have *enough* stomach acid, as opposed to too much. All of our vitamins and minerals need the presence of hydrochloric (HCl) acid in the stomach to be reabsorbed, especially our calcium, magnesium, and Vitamin D. So, when someone tells me they don't have enough calcium, or vitamin D, or that they have osteopenia/osteoporosis, my initial response is not to suggest a calcium supplement; rather, I advise them that they should supplement with some HCl first, then assess if there is still a calcium deficiency.

How does someone become deficient in HCl? The body makes its own HCl, but as we age, our bodies don't produce as much of it. Medications and mental/emotional stresses will suppress the body from releasing its own. Fast food, fried food, packaged and processed foods, and sugars will have the same effect, as will grains and animal products like meats and dairy. If the actual scenario is that you didn't have enough stomach acid and then were given an antacid, you have just lowered the level of stomach acid even more!

In summary, hydrochloric acid is a vital digestive compound that supports the digestive process. With the symptoms for too much stomach acid and not enough stomach acid being basically the same, taking an antacid may reduce low stomach acid even more. The majority of people don't have enough stomach acid, yet many are treated as having too much.

The next stop? The small intestine.

The Truth about the Small Intestine

Even before the food leaves the stomach, the pancreas releases digestive enzymes into the small intestine to get ready for its major role: breaking foods down into separate nutrients. There are different enzymes to break down the proteins, fats, carbohydrates and sugars. Once these macronutrients are broken down into separate vitamins and minerals, they are reabsorbed into the bloodstream through the lining of the small intestine. The blood carries any waste (anything that is *not* of value to the body) to the liver. The liver then "sorts the laundry" sending the body's waste to be eliminated through four main mechanisms—the kidneys, skin, lungs, and colon. If you didn't get all of that, don't worry—there won't be a test!

Let's do a quick review: Fifty percent of the body's waste should be eliminated through the kidneys, 25 percent through the skin, 23 percent through the lungs and only 2 percent through the colon. As I mentioned earlier, all four of these mechanisms, however, need water in order for the body's waste to be eliminated. Otherwise, the toxins and waste are staying in us, causing inflammation. Remember to drink half of your body weight in ounces of water each day at a minimum, and don't drink liquids (water or anything else) with your meals, so the digestive enzymes are not diluted.

How can the small intestine not function properly? First, if the food isn't broken down well enough in the stomach (because of lack of hydrochloric acid for example), then it is passed on to the small intestine only partially digested. The partially digested foods start poking holes into the lining of the small intestine, allowing protein molecules to get reabsorbed into the bloodstream. This may cause hidden food sensitivities, which could lead to a host of other health problems including autoimmune diseases and inflammation in general.

I will cover hidden food sensitivities later, but for now let me tell you about three huge culprits to a lot of digestive problems: gluten, cow's milk (including ice cream), and sugar. When we combine all three of these together, we are headed down the path of disease for ourselves and our children. Think about how most Americans, including children, start their day; often it is with a big bowl of gluten-laden cereal, with cow's milk poured on top (it doesn't matter if it is 2 percent, 1 percent or nonfat—milk is milk!) and a heaping spoonful (or two!) of sugar. They've just had all three major food culprits that cause digestive problems (and a host of other health problems) to start their day—probably every day. With 70 percent of our immune system in the gut, it may not be exposure to other kids at school that is making our children sick—it could be their food! More specifically, food which causes the digestive system to be very much out of balance. This is the type of breakfast children are given by the schools too. Such a diet also contributes heavily to the ADD and ADHD diagnoses we see in our children. Instead of addressing their poor diets, they are routinely given Schedule II controlled drugs like Ritalin and others—the same classification of drug that substances like fentanyl and oxycontin are in.

See https://americanaddictioncenters.org/prescription-drugs/classifications for more information on these drugs. We need to look at the side effects of these drugs on children and rethink how we look at feeding our families. Once again, I digress.

So how do you protect the small intestine? Start by eating real food—not packaged/processed foods, sugars, etc.—avoid foods that are inflammatory and load up on the noninflammatory foods. Next, be sure that your stomach is getting enough stomach acid, and then supplement each of your meals with a broad scope, quality digestive enzyme (not a synthetic one from the discount department store or other similar source). This will help ensure that the food is being broken down properly in order for the nutrients to be reabsorbed.

By now, you are likely starting to notice how the body works as a whole from just this small glimpse. If the stomach doesn't work well, there will be an impact on the small intestine. If the pancreas isn't able to release the digestive enzymes properly because it has been overworked dealing with things like excessive sugar and diabetes, then it too is having a negative impact on our digestive system. The solution to health problems is not to address the symptom, the disease, or the organ that is in a state of "dis-ease," by cutting it out. The key is to treat the person as a whole, and balance the internal environment of the body, starting with the digestive system.

Next, we will continue with the digestive system, focusing on the large intestine and how when it's healthy it can lead to a much greater opportunity for the rest of the body to be healthy too.

The Truth about the Large Intestine

We have been talking about the importance of the digestive system to our overall health. If the digestive system is not functioning properly, we are going to have a hard time achieving optimum health and healing in any other area of our body. To achieve health using natural approaches, the digestive system *must* function optimally. So far, we have talked about the stomach and the need for enough hydrochloric acid, as well as the small intestine and the importance of digestive enzymes and avoiding the inflammatory foods. Next, let's talk about the third major organ of the digestive system, the large intestine, otherwise known as the colon.

The two main functions of the large intestines are to reabsorb the water into the cells where it is needed most, and to store the fecal matter for elimination. There is that need for water again! Since 2 percent of the body's waste *should* be eliminated through the colon, it needs enough water to be able to do this.

Seventy percent of the immune system is in the gut, so it is imperative that it be healthy. Trillions of live, good bacteria reside in the colon—or at least there should be. Yet when we eat the Standard American Diet (SAD), take medications (especially antibiotics), are stressed, consume foods we are sensitive to, and don't have daily bowel movements, our colon becomes overtaken with *bad* bacteria. This is what opens the doors to a multitude of health problems, including cancer—not only in the colon but elsewhere.

Our colon is like the garbage can of our bodies. If the garbage (i.e., the fecal matter) doesn't get taken out on a regular basis, it can sit in the steamy hot environment of our colon for days. The garbage will start to ferment (mainly the carbohydrates/sugars), putrefy (the proteins), and go rancid (the fats). This is what happens in our bodies when we don't have daily bowel movements, enough hydrochloric acid in our stomachs, or enough digestive enzymes to break down the foods. The end result is a toxic body, with inflammation, a multitude of symptoms, and disease. These symptoms and diseases can be endless and we've covered them already; the bottom line is when you have a very dirty garbage can inside of you, you will be sick.

If you are constipated, the first thing to consider is whether you are drinking enough water. If not, the body is robbing the water from the colon for the needs of the cells, leaving the colon dry and thus constipated. This environment is the breeding ground for bad bacteria to occur. Even if we think we are having good, daily bowel movements, that bad bacteria can still grow. That is why it is very important to take a *quality* probiotic as part of our ongoing daily supplement regimen. If you have any kind of gut issues or are on antibiotics, you especially should be taking a high-quality probiotic to restore the good bacteria our bodies desperately need.

In addition to the need for sufficient water and probiotics, fiber from *real foods* like fruits, leafy green vegetables, sweet potatoes and squash, ground flax seed, chia seeds, nuts, etc., is also important.

If you must take a fiber supplement, be sure it is high quality. Do NOT take fiber replacements, stool softeners, and other similar options you might find at the discount stores and drugstores. These can actually cause the colon to become dependent and eventually it may not function properly on its own. The colon is a muscle that needs to be strengthened; using commercial products may cause the colon to weaken. Look for a product with high-quality psyllium fiber in it and avoid those that contain senna.

The good bacteria will eat up the bad bacteria. A quality probiotic has to have live cultures in it, or you will be defeating your purpose in taking one.

As mentioned above, if you are taking an antibiotic, you especially need a high potency, quality probiotic. Antibiotics not only kill the bad bacteria, but they kill the good bacteria too. Your body is left even more vulnerable by taking an antibiotic than it was to start. That's why yeast infections, colds, and other health problems seem to follow antibiotic use. Yes, there is a time and place for antibiotics, but they are being way, way over prescribed.

If you only have finances in your budget for one supplement, I would start with a quality probiotic. I believe it is even more vital to our health than a good multivitamin, because if our digestive system is not functioning properly, it will have a hard time assimilating and utilizing those vitamins and minerals and certainly any nutritional foods you feed it. We always want to support our digestive system so it can then protect all the other areas of our body—after all, it is 70 percent of our immune system!

Most commercial yogurts do not offer live strains of probiotics, in addition, they also contain the sugar or artificial sweeteners that contributed to the problem in the first place. Fermented products such as organic yogurt and kefir that have no sugar are okay, but I do not believe they are the best sources of the probiotics our bodies need. Be sure that live cultures are put back in by the manufacturer after the processing of these foods; it should say somewhere on the packaging that this has been done. With over 2,000 different strains of good bacteria, yogurt simply isn't enough.

NOTE: Probiotics should be taken at bedtime, after the digestive system is done doing its work for the day. There are also quality probiotics that are "shelf-stable," meaning they don't need to be refrigerated. Either type is fine; those that require refrigeration and those that don't.

In summary, drink plenty of water every day, eat lots of fiber-rich foods, and take a quality probiotic supplement. This will give you a "happy" colon and a healthy body.

As a recap, here are some foundational supplements to assist the digestive system in functioning optimally: HCl for the stomach, a good digestive enzyme for the small intestine, and a quality probiotic for the colon. The HCl and digestive enzymes should *only* be taken with meals, while the best time to take the probiotic is at bedtime, once the digestive system is done doing its work for the day.

A Quick Word about the Gallbladder

The gallbladder's responsibility is to break down the fats that are consumed by the body, whether they are good or bad fats. God did not make any other organ in the body to break down the fat; if your gallbladder is removed, your body is compromised for the rest of your life. Because the gallbladder works very closely with the liver, once it is removed the liver compensates by trying to handle the fats that are passing through it. Since the liver wasn't made for that function, it too starts to be compromised. As a result, the liver can develop a condition known as a "fatty congested liver," and an adverse cascade effect begins.

There is a simple gallbladder flush that can maintain or restore the health of the gallbladder. I once had a patient who went to her medical doctor with complaints of gut pain. He felt certain it was her gallbladder and scheduled her first for an ultrasound to confirm his diagnosis, and then to remove it. Fortunately, she came in to see me before the ultrasound and told me about her medical visit. I told her about the gallbladder flush, which she went home and did. Immediately following the flush, her symptoms were about 80 percent better, and within a day or two, gone all together. She then went for her scheduled ultrasound and the report was "unremarkable," meaning no gallstones were evident. Thank you, Jesus! I feel confident if she had not done the gallbladder flush, she would now be walking around without a gallbladder and with her health forever compromised.

See Dr. Hulda Clark's protocol at https://drclark.net/en-us/cleanses/liver-cleanse-page/liver-cleanse-recipe2 to learn more. I do this twice a year, just as routine maintenance of the gallbladder. I have never had gallbladder symptoms and yet I get stones and sludge out every single time—it's amazing!

Note: You can still benefit from this gallbladder flush even if your gallbladder has been removed. In most cases what is known as the "biliary tree" (the various ducts that go to the gallbladder) remains and stones and sludge can accumulate here as well.

We have been talking about the various parts of the digestive system and the very important roles that each plays in obtaining and maintaining optimum health. This system of the body cannot be overlooked if we want to reverse the chronic and degenerative diseases so many people are walking around with these days. This is one of four organs or systems of the body that I believe we can tie almost all chronic and degenerative diseases back to if they are out of balance. Remember, if you want to approach your health wholistically and naturally, one of our main objectives is to get to the *root cause* of the problem, using natural approaches. Next, I would like to talk about the last of these four major organs/systems—the gut/brain connection.

Truth about the Gut/Brain Connection

If you haven't picked up on this by now, let me say it again, our body works as a whole—all the parts are connected and interrelated and have an influence, whether good or bad, on each other. No organ or system of the body works independently of the others. The Bible says this exact thing in 1 Corinthians 12, that is, all of the parts of the body (meaning the Body of Christ) are important, and we can't function without each other; this analogy applies to our literal bodies as well. This leads us into the fourth organ that I feel plays a very foundational role in our overall health—the brain. More specifically, the gut/brain axis or connection plays a huge role in whether the body is healthy or not. There is a cranial nerve that goes from the base of the brain down to the gut, called the vagus nerve. If this nerve is severed, all kinds of bodily functions are disrupted, including many functions of the digestive system.

Remember, 70 percent of the immune system is in the gut. The digestive system is now referred to as the body's "second brain." The digestive system actually has its own nervous system, called the enteric nervous system, and communicates with the brain through the vagus nerve. There certainly is direct communication and influence from the gut to the brain and the brain to the gut. If the digestive system is unhealthy, there is no question that the brain is as well, and all the functions it performs are affected. If the brain is unhealthy i.e.., decline in memory or learning, emotions out of balance, and all the other myriad functions the brain performs—look to the gut first. If there is inflammation in the gut, there is inflammation in the brain causing a state of disease or dysfunction for the brain.

Seventy percent of both women's and men's estrogen is made in the gut. One of the many, many functions of the brain is to regulate our brain chemicals, otherwise known as neurotransmitters—including serotonin, dopamine, melatonin, GABA, leptin, ghrelin, and so many more. And of course, these brain chemicals have a multitude of functions—not just regulating our mood and emotions, but our sleep and appetite as well. If there is an imbalance in any of these areas, the gut has to be addressed. As long as the digestive system is not functioning optimally, no number of supplements or worse—drugs—will change the imbalance in the brain.

One More Organ—Our Skin!

I would be remiss if I did not address the largest organ of our body—the skin! In particular, what we put on our skin, including our hair and mouth. The cells that are on the body's outer skin are the same types of cells that line our entire digestive tract—from the mouth and lining of our nasal passages all the way down to the anus.

The skin is the immune system's first line of defense against many foreign invaders. While we might not be able to tie the majority of chronic and degenerative diseases directly to the health of our skin, it can be a huge entry point for a lot of inflammatory offenders if we are not careful.

The skin has the ability to absorb anything we put on it. That's why those who might be on an estrogen or testosterone cream are prescribed for transdermal application (i.e., on the skin) to get it into the body quicker.

There are what is known as "dirty ingredients" and "clean ingredients." Once again, the majority of the products we buy to maintain our daily hygiene and beauty regimens typically come from the drug, grocery, or discount department stores. These products have so many toxic and cancer-causing ingredients in them that are allowed by the FDA, it's scary.

For example, toothpaste, shampoos, body washes, etc.—things that foam—have an ingredient called sodium lauryl sulfate (SLS), that along with parabens (a type of wax) and aluminum (commonly used in deodorants and sunscreens) are toxic to our bodies. The irony about most sunscreens is they are formulated with cancer-causing ingredients to keep out the sun, which is blamed for causing skin cancer! They also screen out the main natural source of Vitamin D, which is an immune booster. It's like having a mammogram that uses radiation that causes cancer to make sure you don't have cancer. Remember we talked about "Truth is Common Sense Simple?!"

I could write a whole book on all the dirty ingredients included in our beauty products like makeup and lipstick, and in a myriad of conventional products, but others have already done so. See my resource page at the end of the book for a few recommendations.

The good news is there are healthy alternatives to all of these products. Yes, you may pay a little more, but remember that your health is no place to pinch pennies! The important thing is that you are aware of these dirty ingredients now and can make changes to the products you use today!

Call to Action: In summary, there are four organs or systems of the body that are what I call the "heavy hitters." That is, the majority of our chronic degenerative imbalances and diseases can be traced back to at least one of them as the root.

Whether you are closer to the left end of the spectrum of health or have been diagnosed with a disease, in which of the four organs/systems do you think your root cause might lie? I encourage you to consider this carefully and begin healing that organ or system. Perhaps you will start with a liver detox or by taking some supplements for your digestive health. You might also assess the stressors in your life—chemical, mental/emotional, and physical. How can you start reducing that stress? Remember that stress, inflammation, acidic pH, and toxic are four words that are "interchangeable"—if one is there, the others are there. Minimize the stresses and you will minimize the inflammation.

Set a goal and develop some action steps to tackle the area you want to heal first. Take one step at time; even baby steps are steps in the right direction. Remember that your health *is* in your control!

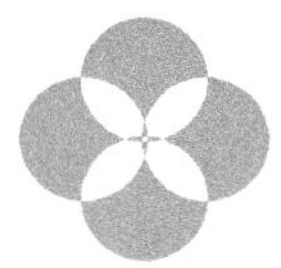

CHAPTER 8

The Connection Between Trauma & Addiction or "Which Came First, The Chicken or The Egg?" (*Stress or Addiction?*)

"The Spirit of the Lord GOD is upon me; because the LORD hath anointed me to preach good tidings unto the meek; he hath sent me to bind up the brokenhearted, to proclaim liberty to the captives, and the opening of the prison to them that are bound."

—Isaiah 61:1 NKJV

Let's pause, back up, and take another big picture look at wholistic health and how an imbalance in our health as a whole can have a negative impact on our mental/emotional state.

Here are some things to review:

- Our health is wholistic—interconnected and related: mental, emotional, physical, and spiritual. None of these can function—whether good or bad—without having an influence on the other areas of our health.
- By mental health I mean time management, budget, career, goal setting, *our purpose in life*—i.e., do we even know why we get out of bed in the morning and what the point is?
- The spiritual and emotional are very closely tied together. In its simplest sense, the good emotions are from God and the bad emotions are from the enemy.
- Within the physical quadrant of the health pie there are five pieces that are vital and foundational to any one of us achieving and maintaining optimum health and healing: rest, water, exercise, good nutrition in and toxins eliminated, and good nerve supply.
- Four words are interchangeable: Stress <> Inflammation <> Acidic <> Toxic—if one is there, the others are there too.
- Three kinds of stress: mental/emotional, chemical, and physical.
- The adrenal glands release a hormone called cortisol that acts as the body's natural anti-inflammatory, responding to all stresses and inflammation.

Now let's take a look at trauma, which is a major mental/emotional, and even spiritual, stressor to the body. Know this: Trauma=Stress, and Stress=Inflammation=Toxic. Drugs—whether prescription or street—are very toxic to the body. In the most basic sense, you are likely able to see the common denominators here.

These words are interchangeable. Things like mental, emotional, physical, verbal and sexual abuse are 100 percent trauma—and they are also 100 percent stress.

While we are talking about emotional health and trauma, will you indulge me for a minute and take a little trip down a short rabbit trail with me? That is, down the trail of "addiction." I feel like this condition is too prevalent in our society these days to be ignored. While we might first think of drugs or alcohol when we hear the word addiction—and it definitely is a huge problem in our society today that is sadly only getting worse—there are other addictions as well; it really can be to just about anything. I recommend reading this information from a wholistic perspective—looking at it from all angles—the mental, emotional, physical, and spiritual. At the same time, keep in mind that trauma is stress and stress is inflammation. Addiction quite often stems from trauma, and addiction is stressful to the body.

I'd like to share a few traumatic stories with you. In fact, these stories are far more common than most people care to admit—it's sometimes easier to put on our rose-colored glasses and then stick our heads in the sand.

Diana's Story

Diana was sexually abused by her natural father for years as a young girl. As she grew into a teenager, she started "looking for love in all the wrong places." Every young man she hooked up with introduced her to yet a different mood-altering drug. You see, when abuse—of any kind—takes place, quite often the default is to either lash out and rebel, or to stuff it down and hide within oneself. Meanwhile, the stress on the body continues. One day, she learned her father committed suicide. This was enough trauma in her life to send her over the edge. She prepared to commit suicide to the point that she was actually sitting over the railing of a bridge that crossed over the interstate, ready to jump and end her life. Fortunately, she had a praying mama. In Diana's case, the trauma/stress came first, then the addiction.

Joan's Story

For another young lady, family life was good. She was raised in a good Christian home, but she was led by the peer pressure of her classmates to "just try it"—the "it" was a very addictive drug. All it took for her body was "just once," and she was hooked. This was also stressful for the body. The addiction came first, leading to stress and trauma.

And one more story:

Nancy's Story

Nancy experienced a traumatic childhood, was abused, addicted to heroin and cocaine, experienced homelessness, lost custody of her three children, attempted suicide multiple times, and had guns pointed at her head. She woke up in an abandoned house, hearing rats crawling in the walls, and discovered her friend lying next to her—dead. She shot up with her friend's dope first before calling the police. At 3:00 a.m. one morning she was sitting in a church parking lot with drugs, money, and a gun feeling a strong spiritual presence in a battle between good and evil—and wondering who would win.

As many as 80 percent of women seeking treatment for drug abuse report life histories of sexual and/or physical abuse. A lot of the time this has occurred as children and at the hands of their protectors.

Trauma = Stress

Along with Post-Traumatic Stress Disorder (make no mistake—abuse victims suffer from PTSD) can come substance abuse, psychiatric issues, pain, sleep problems, cognitive symptoms, medical conditions, relationship problems, etc.

As the number of traumatic events experienced during childhood increases, the risk for the following health problems in adulthood increases:

- depression
- suicide attempts
- alcoholism
- heart and liver diseases
- drug abuse
- pregnancy problems
- high stress
- uncontrollable anger
- family, financial, and job problems

Trauma can cause actual physical changes to the brain. Think of physical and emotional trauma as extreme stress, and the physiological impact on the body. Researchers have found that people who suffer from chronic trauma—for example from childhood abuse—actually have a smaller hippocampus, an area in the brain that is involved in verbal declarative memory. Having a smaller hippocampus may contribute to difficulties with learning and memory.

Two of the brain's functions that are most affected by trauma are learning and physical and mental health. Cortisol and norepinephrine play a critical role in the stress response ("fight or flight") and also have an essential role in memory, showing the important link between learning, memory, and the body's traumatic stress response. Trauma also impacts physical and mental health as the stress of trauma leads to anxiety, depression, PTSD, a multitude of health issues including chronic inflammation, digestive and autoimmune disorders, cancers, and heart disease.

After...*The Wholistic Approach*

As of my writing this book, Diana is thriving in her workplace where she has been for over five years now. Her relationship with her mom is amazing and she is now a solid mother to her own daughter, who is quickly growing into a young healthy woman.

Joan is just a little ball of energy, and it is quite apparent God's hand and favor is upon her life! She keeps advancing in the business world from the manufacturing floor, driving a forklift to administrative work in a highly respected corporation in her town. She loves Jesus and it shows!

Nancy has been free and clean from her addictions for almost six years now. She surrounds herself with positive influences in her life and regularly attends peer support group meetings. She has worked her way up the ladder in a manufacturing business, from laborer to administrative work—and is still moving up. The center of her life is a life in Jesus Christ. She finds peace, love, and joy in this life. To see the glow on her face these days is to know she maintains a healthy diet. She is still working on obtaining visitation rights with her three children. All three of these ladies, and many more, have a brand-new life, thanks to living it wholistically!

The combination of scenarios can go on and on. The point is that it doesn't really matter whether trauma or addiction came first.

There is more to addiction than some teenager wanting to rebel and be cool. It is a full-blown disease like any other. Similarly, the body *can* most effectively be restored to good health and set free from diseases, including addiction, that bind them when they are addressed from a wholistic approach.

Call to action: ask yourself what you are addicted to. Did you experience any traumas in your life, especially as a child? A word of caution and encouragement here: what you might not think was a trauma could very well have been. Don't dismiss the harmful things that have happened in your life—even if it was the fault of no one.

Perhaps your house caught on fire, you were in a bad car accident, you had a very frightful scare when a dog attacked you as a child. The possibilities are endless. Give thought to these things and address them. Perhaps seek some counseling, or at the very least share it with a trusted friend, family member, spouse, or minister. Please don't underestimate the influence this or other multiple traumas can have on the challenges you face in overcoming your health problems.

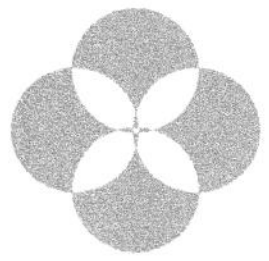

SECTION 3

Truth vs. Deception: Live a Life of Health and Empowerment!

As the years go by, my eyes continue to be opened to more and more confusions, myths and deceptions as it pertains to folks understanding the endless possibilities for their health to be restored, as those possibilities are tremendously over-shadowed by the paradigm of disease management rather than health restoration.

I probably could write an entire book on each of these myths and deceptions, but for now I will briefly share some additional enlightenments in this section as to how you can restore your health when viewed from a wholistic perspective. We'll also revisit some of the information we have already addressed, but in a little more depth, with the hopes of bringing a little more clarity to some of the things I have already shared with you.

And hopefully some of the information will cause you to simply pause and ponder a moment—and perhaps bring you back to a place of common-sense awareness of how the traditional approaches of disease management have been presented to us with what is being called "health."

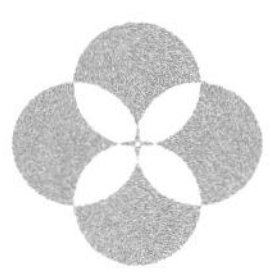

CHAPTER 9

The Truths: Open Your Eyes and Ears!

"Do not be deceived, my beloved brothers and sisters. Every good thing given and every perfect gift is from above, coming down from the Father of lights, with whom there is no variation or shifting shadow."

—James 1:16-17 NASB

This next section is to summarize the presented information and share a collection of some other misperceptions or deceptions about true wholistic health and wellness.

Root Cause vs. Disease Management

We covered this topic at the beginning of the book, but it is certainly worth repeating. True wholistic health and wellness are about getting to the root cause of the problem and then working toward restoring the body to good health. These are the two primary objectives of wholistic health and wellness.

For a century or more, we have been bombarded by the traditional medical practice of looking at a symptom, isolating that symptom as if it did not have any impact on the rest of the body, and basically then just addressing that one symptom. This is the method that continues to be used, whether it's a lab value showing too high or too low, a pain somewhere, or any other number of symptoms such as fatigue, headache, joint pain, and gut pain. The eventual outcome, or solution is to take a pill—usually a prescribed medication—to make the symptom go away or have the lab numbers return to within a normal reference range. This is not health: This is only management of the disease. True wholistic health treats the entire patient.

Nutrition vs. Calories

I once presented a Truth About Wellness workshop to a Parent-Teacher Association (PTA) meeting at an elementary school where I was a business partner. My hope was to do monthly workshops for the parents just prior to their PTA meetings. A day or so after my initial presentation, I received a fairly demanding call from a woman who had attended that meeting. Identifying herself by just her first name, and as a parent, she wanted to know what authority I had to speak about foods that are good for us and those that are not. After about 10 minutes of interrogation by this arrogant woman, she revealed to me that she was a dietician and stated, "only dieticians have the 'legal' right to tell people what they can eat!" I kid you not, she really said that! I then told her I was curious as to why dieticians feed hospitalized diabetic patients a diet of pastas, breads, and even desserts. Her simple, nothing more-nothing less answer was "well they need their calories."

OK then... This was a tremendous eye opener for me, and confirmation that there is nothing more important to them than calories when it comes to diet. It doesn't matter what those calories are made up of, or that they can actually be harming the patient instead of helping—they just want to make sure you get those calories, no matter the cost—whether it's your health or even your life. This was just the first time I heard this defense, but I have heard it many more times in the years that followed. Recall how I shared earlier the story of my sister-in-law being fed donuts during her chemo treatments? Outrageous.

In reality, our health and the foods we eat or don't eat should be measured by the nutrients we are needing, lacking, and/or taking in, as well as the toxic ingredients we are consuming that make up those calories.

Nutritionist vs. Dietician

When any one of us starts treating ourselves through the advice of "Dr. Internet," it can be a good thing, and it can be a bad thing—and usually it's a little of both! What is to be commended is that the first step toward restoring the body back to good health is admitting that there is something out of balance to begin with and wanting to do something about it. The bad thing is that there is so much conflicting information out there that it can make our heads spin, and then we throw up our hands and put our heads back in the sand to deal with it another day.

The other important point I want to make is the difference between a dietician and a (true) nutritionist.

> *According to Wikipedia, "Founded in 1917 as the American Dietetic Association, the organization officially changed its name to the Academy of Nutrition and Dietetics in 2012." Again, from Wikipedia, "A licensed nutritionist is a professional who has earned credentials through a nationally recognized licensing body. These include the Commission on Dietetic Registration (CDR), the Board for Certification of Nutrition Specialists (BCNS), and the Clinical Nutrition Certification Board (CNCB)."*

Prior to 2012, you could easily tell if the source of health information you were reading was coming from a dietician (i.e., the medical profession, since dieticians are licensed as such), or from an independent nutritionist, licensed under their own board, simply by their title or organization name (Dietician or Nutritionist). Unfortunately, requirements vary by state, and not all fifty states recognize nutritionists that are not licensed under the medical board. Also unfortunate is that the dieticians' association hijacked the title nutritionist so you can't tell the difference as to which camp the nutritionist truly belongs to, at least not very easily. You must read between the lines a little more now.

Regardless of title, though, you will always want to first check your source of the health information you are researching before pursuing any advice. Second, you should research the motivation behind the information. Is it for the purpose of selling you their brand of supplement or their services, or are they truly wanting to impart their God-given gift to help you achieve greater wholistic health? Lastly, check that their philosophy and objectives are in line with yours. Are they about managing disease or getting to the root cause?

The important thing is that *you* know there is a big difference between a dietician and a true wholistic nutritionist.

The Truth about Supplements

When I was in chiropractic school, just learning about the whole natural health topic, I was having some major digestive issues going on—the irritable bowel syndrome from childhood was rearing its ugly head in full force! I went to the local health food store and inquired with the clerk as to what was good for a digestive problem; with confidence she suggested Aloe Vera juice. I bought it with the belief this was going to be the "cure" for what ailed me. Not so much. That incident became a learning lesson for me.

First of all, remember, "there is no magic pill." There typically is not just one thing that causes an issue, and there almost always is not just one thing that cures it. Hopefully, by this point in the book, you will understand that. It's really about getting to the root cause of the problem and not just addressing the symptoms. That's why when asked "What should I take for…" my standard response is, "I don't know; I don't know what's causing your symptoms, problem, etc."

An important lesson about supplements is there is a huge difference between your mass-marketed retail products and quality supplements. Having worked in a health food store, I learned what those differences are.

While working in the natural products industry, I had the opportunity to train under the owner of Gaia Herbs Farms, a high-quality organic supplement company. Their main farm and office are in Brevard, North Carolina. The owner would offer an all-day tour of their gorgeous organic herbal farm and provide a beautiful healthy lunch to health-food store employees, nutritionists, and others. I learned so much from this man and their quality manufacturing processes. That's not to say that only Gaia Herbs follows manufacturing best practices; there are many other quality supplement companies out there too.

Even better than quality retail products are the quality practitioner/professional line of supplements, otherwise known as nutraceuticals. Gaia Herbs is both professional and retail. One of the practices of both quality retail and professional nutraceutical companies is to participate in a voluntary third-party verification. Of the many criteria for this, is that the raw ingredients they say are in their products truly are in there. The other thing that sets quality supplements apart from mass-produced products is the source and purity of their raw materials. Very high-tech machines test samples to meet stringent requirements, and if any impurities are found (like trace heavy metals), the batch is automatically rejected.

Quality supplement manufacturers harvest their ingredients differently than those in mass production. I always like to use herbs as an example of this. Let's say you wanted to take some echinacea for a cold you feel may be coming on. You go to the discount department store because it's cheaper and you think to yourself, "It's all the same, let me just buy the cheapest (or even mid-priced) product because you get what you pay for, right?" However, the difference between the echinacea from the discount store and one from a quality supplier is that the discount brand uses the flower of the plant instead of the root of the plant. Yet it's the *root* of the plant that contains the healing properties you are looking for to calm that cold. The flower has no healing properties, but it's still echinacea. Therein lies the difference in how the ingredients are harvested and used.

One last, and very important point, regarding herbs in particular. A mass-produced, cheap herb sold at the discount store could have been harvested three times from the same field during one growing season, thereby losing its nutritional value as well as its efficacy because it was picked too early or too late—possibly in soil that was depleted of vital nutrients.

Also, the vitamins found in discount stores, drug stores, and grocery stores are usually synthetically produced. They are made to mimic the real vitamin; however, the problem is that it's not real, and no vitamin or mineral is found all by itself in nature. It needs the other vitamins and minerals to function as it was designed by God to do. Almost always, formulas are better, whether mass produced or quality manufactured.

Allergies vs. Hidden Food Sensitivities

Did you know there is a difference between "allergies" and "hidden food sensitivities?" There is, in fact, a BIG difference. Most people don't realize this and probably, for whatever reason, most allergists don't acknowledge it. Allergies are the focus for traditional medical doctors, ignoring the adverse effects of hidden food sensitivities.

The immune system has five different types of immunoglobulins—IgA, IgE, IgG, IgM, and IgD—each performing different important functions for the body. For example, IgA protects the mucous membrane layers in the body, including the lining of the mouth, gut, and entire digestive tract. IgE provides an immediate response to allergens; this is what an allergist typically tests. For example, if you've ever broken out in hives from eating peanuts or reacted severely to a bee sting, this is a histamine response that activates the IgE immunoglobulin. If someone is having allergy symptoms, they may go to an allergist who will do a "pin prick" or "scratch test" to assess all kinds of different allergens. These are the tests done for an "immediate response" to an allergen.

What doctors don't seem to give much credence to, and therefore don't often test, is the IgG immunoglobulin. IgG is the most common and abundant antibody present in the body. Blood plasma consists of 75-80 percent of IgG antibodies. Of all antibodies, IgG has the longest lifespan of about 23 days. IgG is the only antibody that can cross the placental barrier and provide passive immunity to a developing fetus. Seems pretty significant to me!

IgG immunoglobulin will present with a delayed response to hidden food sensitivities. This means you could eat an apple today and as many as 3 days later present with any number of symptoms. You would not likely associate the apple you ate 3 days ago with the headache you are experiencing today. To make matters worse, you know that "an apple a day keeps the doctor away," so you eat an apple every day, thereby creating a chronic headache. The symptoms truly can be endless when we are consuming hidden food sensitivities—anything from gut, skin, and joint issues to even emotional responses.

When we consume foods we are sensitive to, the body experiences inflammation which can then cause adverse chemical reactions in the body. Remember:

Stress = Inflammation = Acidic = Toxic

The proteins of these foods cause the immune system to respond, and when we consume them, they start poking holes in the lining of the gut. This allows the proteins to escape into the bloodstream, wreaking all kinds of havoc in any number of places in the body.

If someone is being challenged with autoimmune conditions, one of the first things a functional medicine doctor will tell the patient to do is avoid gluten, dairy, and sugar—three categories of foods that cause an extremely high inflammatory response. In fact, cow's milk is the leading hidden food sensitivity, it is very inflammatory and very mucus forming. I can't tell you how many conversations I have had with patients and customers that would come into the health food stores where I worked who would tell me once they stopped drinking cow's milk all of their joint pain went away!

The other tool that is quite common for functional medicine practitioners is a hidden food sensitivity test. They usually test anywhere from 100-250 different hidden foods, spices, and ingredients, and the majority of the foods that are being tested are real and healthy foods that you wouldn't expect to be "bad" for you. For most people they are not, but *your* body might be sensitive to them. I routinely ran a hidden food sensitivity test on patients that checked the top 96 most-common hidden food sensitivities, and it was not uncommon for someone to be sensitive to 20 or more foods.

People are often disappointed when their favorite foods show up on the sensitivity list. The good news is that, in most cases, you can be freed from these sensitivities by avoiding them for a certain time, depending on how sensitive you are to them. Also, you may very well have an IgE (immediate) response to something but not the IgG (delayed) response, or vice versa. This is why it is wise to at least be checked for hidden food sensitivities. To me, the delayed response (IgG) is harder to detect than the immediate response (IgE) when the scratch test or pin prick test is performed. Trust me, if you are allergic (IgE) to peanuts you will know soon enough! With a delayed response, it is not as easy to tell right off hand. Again, the main concern with consuming foods you are sensitive to is that it causes inflammation in the body. This is the primary reason for testing.

Why Are Sodas Dangerous?

I did a workshop once on goal setting and asked the employees to write down some goals. One gal wanted to "cut down" on drinking Mountain Dew but stated that she "loved it!"

Can you see several things wrong with this last sentence? When setting goals (or in anything else we do), it is imperative that we watch the words we speak out loud for "…out of the abundance of his heart, the mouth speaks" (Luke 6:45 NKJV). She stated that she "loved it." This is contrary to her goal, because giving up something that is "loved" means she may not be successful in achieving it.

The next thing that was wrong with this statement is "cut down." If you have been addicted to something, as I have, you know there is no such thing as "cutting down" or "cutting back"—it just isn't going to happen. Oh yes, maybe for a little while, but in the long run with an addiction, you'll be back because it's all or nothing. How did I know she was addicted? I was *there,* I saw the look in her eyes, and the passion in her voice when she said how much she *loved* Mountain Dew! Plus, It's MOUNTAIN DEW, how could she *not* be addicted?! Which leads me into my third point…

Mountain Dew, or any soda for that matter, is dangerous. There truly is no other way to say it—I cannot afford to say it kindly or politically correct—it is poison, and it is very, very toxic. All sodas are—regardless if it's light colored, dark colored, caffeine free, sugar free, whatever—dangerous. I searched the internet for this article "How dangerous is Mountain Dew?" I couldn't count all the links that came up; I would have been there for days if I tried reading all that information. Let me summarize it for you:

The biggest problem with all sodas is that they contain High Fructose Corn Syrup (HFCS). This synthetic sugar is directly linked to obesity, diabetes, high blood pressure, cancer, and so much more; and these are *life-threatening* diseases! I shouldn't have to say anything more to convince you to stop drinking all sodas, not just Mountain Dew. The second biggest problem is that the phosphoric acid in all sodas robs your body—quickly—of its many vital nutrients. To compound this, if you are not feeding your body with vital nutrients to begin with, you are assaulting your body with a "double whammy."

Sodas are very acidic to the body. If you are a soda drinker, more than likely you suffer from some kind of digestive problems—acid reflux, gastroesophageal reflux disease, food sensitivities, etc. That's because the sodas suppress the stomach's demand for hydrochloric acid (HCl), leading you to believe that you need "antacids." Remember, the symptoms are the same for too much stomach acid (hence the antacids) and not enough stomach acid; the majority of the time though it's that we don't have enough stomach acid instead of too much. The body also needs HCl in order to reabsorb calcium and Vitamin D as well as other important nutrients. If you are drinking the sodas that suppress the HCl and taking antacids on top of that, you are not getting the vital life-giving nutrients that you need. There are so many other reasons why you should avoid soda, and this information is just the tip of the iceberg.

Please realize what soft drinks are doing to your body, and that of your children and grandchildren. The solution is to drink water; it is so nourishing to the body!

Butter or Margarine?

Once again, my heart was breaking for the misinformed. I was in a grocery store one day, and I happened to overhear a couple who were probably in their 60s comparing the labels of two brands of margarine. "How much cholesterol? How much trans fats? How many calories…" As politely as I could, I invited myself into their conversation by simply stating "butter is better." The woman proceeded to tell me it was for her father and that "they" won't "let" him have butter, and "they" told him to eat margarine instead. I tried to explain to them that what they were holding in their hands wasn't even real food. They said they knew, but "they" said he was supposed to eat margarine, not butter. She continued by saying if it makes him "feel" better he may as well eat it!

Butter is real food, folks. Eating real butter, in moderation, is certainly far better for anyone, but especially those who are ill, than *any* kind of processed, chemical-laden, tub of plastic. I don't care what the ads in magazines tell you. Ideally the butter you eat is organic, but even if it's not, it's still not near as harmful for you as margarine. I can't even say the word without making a funny face. I actually think of margarine as a product of the 60s—outdated. But apparently, it's still selling strong.

Government Dependency

There has obviously been a strong trend in the past decade (or even longer) of America moving in a socialist direction, with its citizens becoming more dependent on the government. Our "sick care" is no exception. Not just by citizens becoming more dependent on the government to pay for their sick care, but also by the drug companies causing people to become more dependent on them.

In turn, the government includes medications in government programs (i.e., Medicaid, Obamacare, Medicare). The medications they manufacture cause the body to become dependent as well as sicker, in turn, causing the body to need even more medications. It's like the drug companies' enticement to become dependent is camouflaged behind government programs.

Make no mistakes about it, our government and the pharmaceutical companies are making billions of dollars by keeping you sick.

I've said before to follow the money. Between deceptive labeling practices by the FDA, to government subsidies, to the big agribusinesses that make genetically modified foods that make us sick, to the big lobbying groups like the big pharmaceutical and food industries that keep us sick for profit—our health is NOT their concern.

Pharmaceutical Industry

Once again, I could write a whole book on the harm that the pharmaceutical industry has caused millions upon millions of people under the guise of "health." There are tons of books out there that are already written on this subject, so I will just share a few statistics here, and give you recommendations where you can learn in greater detail the truths about this industry.

No doubt these numbers have increased tremendously over the past 10+ years, but in 2010 Gary Null wrote in his book *Death by Medicine*:

- The number of people having in-hospital, adverse reactions to prescribed drugs annually: approximately 2.2 million
- The number of unnecessary and/or inappropriate antibiotics prescribed annually: approximately 45 million per year
- The number of unnecessary medical and surgical procedures performed each year: 7.5 million
- The number of people unnecessarily hospitalized each year: 8.9 million
- The total number of deaths caused by conventional medicine is nearly 800,000 per year

To quote Null from his book, "It is now evident that the American medical system is the leading cause of death and injury in the US." Mr. Null cites his sources for his statistics in his book.

Now please hear me: There absolutely is a time and a place for both the medical profession and pharmaceuticals. When I have to have a major dental procedure, I want Novocain. When I broke my leg backpacking, I wanted an orthopedist, not my chiropractor. Even when I had the kidney stone, I opted for the doctor to go in and remove it as opposed to "waiting" for it to happen on its own; I certainly didn't want to find myself backpacking in the wilderness somewhere by myself and a kidney stone decided to pass! In *choosing* to have the doctor do this, I definitely (as toxic as it is) wanted anesthesia before they did the procedure. And thankfully, he gave me a choice--for the procedure, not the anesthesia!

For the majority of the chronic and degenerative diseases, there is almost always a far better alternative to drugs and surgery. Do your research and be an informed consumer. It is Your health, after all.

Who is the Authority on our Health—God or Modern Medicine?

A while back, I saw two heartbreaking stories printed side by side in the newspaper. The first was about a mother and father who were arrested for manslaughter when their 2-year-old son died. Instead of taking him to a medical doctor, they chose to trust in God to heal their son —for this they were convicted and their lives forever changed. I was reminded of a similar situation when a mother was tracked down by the FBI and arrested when she took her son to Mexico for alternative treatment for his cancer. She was accused of child abuse because she didn't take him to a medical doctor for chemotherapy.

Does God still heal and perform miracles today? Absolutely. He is the same yesterday, today, and forever more. Is the medical approach the *only* right approach to cancer treatment? Absolutely not.

There are thousands of testimonies of people healed from all kinds of diseases, including cancers, utilizing natural approaches. Look up Dr. Francisco Contreras with Oasis of Hope in Mexico if you want to learn about some of the many healings.

There is a flip side to the authority story. There have been multiple stories over the years of teenagers committing suicide by setting their bodies on fire. I would bet anything that each of these kids was on some kind of mood-altering prescribed medication—either something for attention deficit, anxiety, depression, or similar. I just can't imagine someone in this state of mind not under psychiatric care, and I certainly can't imagine them not being prescribed drugs. When I read these stories, I was reminded of a very similar situation. Author Gwen Olsen, who is a former pharmaceutical drug rep, was compelled to get out of the business and write her book, *True Confessions of an Rx Drug Pusher* when her niece, who was in her early 20s committed suicide by setting *herself* on fire as well. She started off on prescription medications because of an auto accident. She experienced side effects from the pain medications, with one of those being depression. She was then put on antidepressants which also had side effects. She was then diagnosed as bi-polar and given more medications, followed by a schizophrenia diagnosis and more medications, until eventually she committed suicide. Coincidence? I doubt it.

'Let me ask you this: Why were the parents of the child who died because they trusted God instead of modern medicine convicted of manslaughter? What about the mother who wanted to implement a more natural approach for her child's cancer treatment, instead of a toxic approach like chemotherapy, charged with abuse, but the parents of the teenagers who committed suicide (probably because of side effects from the antidepressants prescribed by modern medicine), *not* arrested and convicted? Now my heart certainly goes out to the parents who have lost children to any form of suicide, and especially something as horrific as setting their bodies on fire. I certainly am not faulting any parent who has their child on antidepressants or any other kind of mood-altering med, as sad as this is to me—that's their choice. Yet my heart equally goes out to parents who choose God or natural approaches for healing for their children and are arrested for doing so. My point is we have a right to make our own choices when it comes to taking care of our children and our own health, whether it be God, natural approaches, or conventional medicine. The government and so-called modern medicine are *not* the ultimate authority—God is.

By the way, there are over 800,000 deaths per year due to modern medicine—including but not limited to surgeries, drug overdoses, reactions, hospital-induced infections and much more. Per YEAR—and hardly ever a criminal conviction.

Death by modern medicine seems to be just an "unfortunate" situation, but death by trusting God is deemed a crime. Since when was modern medicine put above God for healing? When did the government assign modern medicine the ultimate authority on how one takes care of their health, or even their illness, as opposed to a natural approach or God or even one's free right to choose? Meanwhile, it's okay to kill babies before they are born, and that is the choice of the individual, yet when we trust God or a natural means He has provided us, it becomes a crime punishable by law. I just don't get it.

Health Comes from Above, Down, Inside, and Out

I am going to make a statement that is contrary to western medicine's way of thinking, which has molded and formed most people's way of thinking about their health. We touched on this a little bit at the beginning of the book. The statement is this: "Disease is a general condition of one's *internal* environment." It is not the symptoms we feel or see, nor is it an entity that attacks us from somewhere else. In other words, it's the integrity of the internal environments of our bodies—our digestive system in particular, and also the fluids and our immune system—that determine the level of our health. If the internal environment of our body is healthy, then we can be exposed to the germs on the outside and we should not fear "catching" every little thing. Understand that there are *always* going to be bacteria, viruses, fungi, and the like in our external environment, and for that matter, in the internal environment of our body as well. But if our immune system is up to par, they are unable to overcome us.

This concept is not easy to accept, and it's even harder to live by, but it's the truth. We do not need to be over-spraying everything under the sun with some kind of antibacterial cleaning product that is more toxic than the germs it purports to kill. This is where we start stepping into the major overkill (no pun intended!) of sterilizing everything around us. It's being subjected to all of these "antimicrobial" products—hand sanitizers everywhere, cleaning products, etc.—that is causing us to be too sensitive to the germs when they do present themselves. Not to mention the overkill of all the vaccines kids are receiving these days—quite scary actually.

There was an article in the Charleston, South Carolina, "Post & Courier" newspaper one morning with the headline, "Toll on Children Puzzling."[10] The author explained the infamous swine flu "appears to be taking a higher toll on school-age youngsters than on babies and toddlers." This is a classic example of western medi-

10 "Toll on Children Puzzling," The Post & Courier, September 3, 2009

cine's thought process, which is modeled after Louis Pasteur's theory known as the Germ Theory of Disease. It claims that fixed species of *microbes* from an *external* source invade the body and are the first cause of "infectious" disease. This is the opposite of the true physiology of the body.

When I read this article, it was not surprising to me at all that school-age kids (defined as between the ages of 5 through 17) were more susceptible. Why? We need only to take a look at their diets. Sugars are the breeding ground for all kinds of imbalances to the internal environment of the body, not to mention all the packaged and processed foods with the food additives and preservatives, fast foods, and fried foods. This is setting a tremendous stage for disease in our young people as well as adults. *This* is more of the true reason all of us are unhealthy, not just our kids—it's not because we "touched" something. There are also the highly toxic vaccines children are exposed to *before* they ever even enter kindergarten.

Once again, I know I have only touched the tip of the iceberg by what I mean when I say the "internal environment" of your body, so I highly encourage you to study up on this. Read Robert Young's book *Sick and Tired, Reclaim Your Inner Terrain* or his other book *The pH Miracle*. I have referenced these in the Resource section. This will help give you some insight into how you can bring your body back to good health, naturally, and without drugs or surgeries. When you do this, *you* are in control of your health, not the insurance companies, the drug companies, your employer, or the government (Heaven forbid!).

Count the Cost...

As I was taking my supplements one morning, I got to thinking about how much it cost me to maintain my health. I would have to say that it's not overly expensive, and yet I will be honest with you, there is some cost involved. I do take mostly high-quality nutraceutical grade supplements, and almost everything I consume as food is organic. I invested in a moderately-priced yet quality mattress. I buy a good pair of running shoes several times a year and a pair of custom fitted orthotics once every few years. I purchased a water ionizer, and I replace the filter about twice a year. I also invest *time* in my health. I typically exercise on average three times per week, I allow time for enough sleep, and I spend time with the Lord for my spiritual health. I continue to learn and study for both my professional life and my personal life, so I spend time here as well for my mental health. Please understand, this is not about me and how well I take care of my health; it's merely intended as an example of some costs in doing so. Is there room for improvement? Absolutely! Our health is a process.

However, conversations I have with others regarding their health leave me feeling sad sometimes. Too often I hear "I can't afford to eat healthy," or "I can't afford to buy supplements." Some say they can't afford to see a practitioner that would help them restore their health for a variety of other reasons—justified or not. I also quite often hear about not having *time* to exercise, eat right, rest, or spend quality time with the Lord.

I'll pose a few questions for your reflection. How much do you spend on your vehicle? Consider all things: how much do you spend on gas, your car payment, car insurance, and maintenance (e.g., new tires, oil changes, radiator flushes, alignments)? Then there are emergency expenses, including AAA membership, and a savings account for other vehicle emergencies. Now think about the *time* you (or someone else) put into your vehicle. How often do you wash and wax it and how long does it take? How long do you sit and wait while it's being serviced? How much time (and money) do you spend on license and tag renewals? The list could go on and on.

Now the toughest question of all: between *your* health and your *car's* "health," which one gets allotted more time and money? And before you say, "yeah but I *need* my vehicle, it gets me to and from work, without it I would not have any money at all!" or "I couldn't 'live' without my car!" or "that's not even a fair comparison, I *have* to have my car!" Let me ask you this: Do you need your body? If you didn't have a body, could you make a living? Can you *live* without your body? The answers, of course, are obvious. Unfortunately, we don't think in these terms. The unfortunate thing is people truly value their cars much more than their own health.

What is even worse in my opinion is sometimes I think people truly don't believe that they are worth it. They don't slow down long enough to treasure who they really are. Whether you know it or not and believe it or not, you are valued and treasured beyond your wildest imagination, and certainly beyond any material possessions, including your car. Because YOU truly are a precious, precious child of the Most High Living God, Abba, Father! And if you've invited Jesus Christ to take up residency on the inside of your very being, then your body is also the temple of that Most High Living God: You "house" Him on the very inside of you! Stop for a moment and let that sink in—you are *that* valuable! Much more so than any luxury car out there. Believe and receive it and start walking that out!

Are We Enabling Sickness?

Although I may sound harsh, I speak the truth in love. When I hear the government trying to play on our sympathies by telling stories of someone with a terrible disease who couldn't get their health insurance company to pay for it, I wonder if the person cared enough about their own health *before* they got sick? Please don't misunderstand me, I certainly have empathy for someone who is sick, and there certainly are some cases where a person's illness or disease has nothing to do with their health habits (or lack thereof). However, 80 percent of the time, the illness or disease could have been prevented had the person simply known the truth about health and wellness, and then been proactive with their health and taken care of it. I know you may find this hard to believe, but it's the truth. We have been so bombarded and brain-washed into believing that drugs are the answer, but they are not. Remember, Hippocrates said "let food be your medicine and medicine be your food." Poor Hippocrates—he's probably turning over in his grave right now!

Most people won't even follow the most common sense, inexpensive, simplest protocols to take care of their health. I am not a statistics person, but I know in my heart just from all the research I read and learn about that if these simple protocols were followed faithfully, that in and of itself could lower the cost of health care. These basic protocols consist of *regular* exercise, drinking good pure water, eating chemical free fruits and vegetables, getting seven to nine hours of uninterrupted sleep each night, and making sure your body has good nerve supply. These basic protocols are not too expensive!

We live in such a "dependent," fast-paced, "it's somebody else's responsibility," and "it's my right" society that these basic protocols seem foreign to us. Because it's only by you, yourself, doing each of these protocols that good health can occur. No one else can do these things for you.

I will give my sympathy the next time the government tries to play on it, if they have the nerve to ask the person, first, what they did or didn't do to help themselves. I think if someone is going to receive free healthcare at someone else's expense—whether it be us as the tax-paying citizens via the government, the insurance companies, the healthcare provider, or the employer—they need to do something in return first. That is, they need to demonstrate responsibility for and prove they are doing *their part* in taking care of their own health. It's time to wake up, folks, and not enable sickness—and live the truth about health and wellness.

Not Enough Stomach Acid?

We touched on this in chapter 6, but I would like to elaborate a little more on stomach acid. If you find yourself belching, having acid reflux, heartburn, etc., you probably either assume, or have been told by a medical doctor, that you have too much stomach acid (otherwise known as hydrochloric acid) and take an antacid. There are popular over-the-counter options and medications. Perhaps you think drinking milk is the answer because it soothes the burning for you. Most likely, though, you don't have *enough* stomach acid. The fact there is a drug for having too much stomach acid is why we always hear about it. The symptoms of too much and not enough are the same, but actually more people don't have enough stomach acid.

This can be caused by many things. For example, our bodies don't produce as much stomach acid as we age, stress can suppress it, medications can suppress it, eating carbs and proteins, packaged and processed foods, cow's milk, and sugars can all suppress it, too. Simply put, overconsumption of any unhealthy foods can cause reduced stomach acid. One need not be middle-aged either to have this problem; nowadays it's not uncommon in younger persons as well due to their diets. We need stomach acid to break down our food. In addition, all of our vitamins and minerals need the presence of *enough* stomach acid in order to be reabsorbed, especially calcium, vitamin D, and magnesium. Quite often the reason women become osteoporotic is because they don't have *enough* stomach acid, not because they don't get enough calcium.

Hydrochloric acid serves many functions, two of the most basic being:

1. It is the primary digestive juice responsible for breaking down proteins, preparing them for assimilation.
2. It acts as a protective barrier, killing many potentially harmful microorganisms in our food.

When there isn't enough stomach acid to break down food, it comes back up, bringing some stomach acid with it and causing heartburn and even erosion of the esophagus. You may want to try taking some hydrochloric acid tablets with your meals; get one with around 250ml per tablet (you can find this at your natural health food store). Each body is different; to determine how much YOUR body needs, start by taking one tablet with each meal the first day, the second day take two tablets with each meal, the third day three tablets and keep increasing each day like this until you feel a little warm burning sensation in the upper stomach area within 1-2 hours after eating. Don't be surprised if you get up to 6 tablets or more before feeling this. Once you feel the warm burning sensation (or a funny kind of feeling—for me it feels like I've had too much sugar), you back down by one tablet, and that's YOUR dosage. For example, if at 6 tablets you feel that burning sensation, then your dosage is 5 tablets per meal. Do NOT take them unless you are eating.

NOTES: Don't take HCl if you know you have stomach ulcers, as this will irritate the ulcer. When consuming meals that contain little or no protein or starchy carbs, less hydrochloric acid is needed by the stomach to process its contents. Please keep this in mind when using HCl as a supplement and modify your usage accordingly.

This awareness of actually not having enough stomach acid, and the simple remedy to supplement with hydrochloric acid with meals, was one of the greatest "aha" moments for so many customers when I worked in the health food stores. I can't tell you the number of people who noticed almost immediate results when they ditched their "antacid" and started supporting their body instead.

The Truth about Salt

At the beginning of this book, I spoke of going to an urgent care facility for high blood pressure. After going through the routine spiel of exercise and eating right, the doctor then said, "and no salt." I told him I didn't consume table salt (which is devoid of the other minerals our bodies need), but that I use Celtic sea salt. In a very arrogant way he leaned in, and almost whispered in my ear "salt is salt." (I think my BP most likely shot up a few more points!) He then was ready to write me a prescription—the solution to all things related to high blood pressure (regardless of the root cause). Really?! I flat out told him I would not take that prescription and that he could save the ink in his pen. (OK, I didn't really tell him to save the ink in his pen, but I sure thought so!) Why didn't he give any consideration to the fact that I was sitting there in horrific back pain and *that* could very possibly have been the cause of the high blood pressure? Instead, he just wanted to give me a prescription—that I undoubtedly would have for the rest of my life—and tell me not to eat salt.

The point of this story is that our bodies *need* sodium. In fact, it is the largest portion of minerals in the body. But there *is* a difference between your processed bleached out table salt and *real* salt (e.g., Celtic sea salt or Himalayan salt). These salts have all the other minerals like potassium, chloride, and magnesium in the right proportions, so the sodium functions as God designed it to do. My heart just breaks whenever I hear people being conscious about not eating anything with salt in it but not batting an eye at how much sugar and carbs they consume. The truth is we need real salt; it is vital to our body.

For a true eye opener on how vital salt is, read Dr. David Brownstein's book *Salt Your Way to Health*, listed in the reference section.

Call to Action: There are a number of hidden truths I have called out in this chapter. For two of these I encourage you to take action. First, seek out a functional medicine practitioner who will run a hidden food sensitivity test on you to identify the foods you are sensitive to. If running this test is not in your budget at the moment, or there is not a practitioner in your area, then start by eliminating the most common and highest sensitivity foods: cow's milk/dairy, gluten/wheat, sugar, and possibly eggs. Although eggs are good for you, a fair number of people have a tendency to build up an intolerance to them.

Second, I suggest you peruse the quality, source, and brand of supplements you are taking. If you are taking supplements (and you should at least be taking the foundational ones) that you currently buy from the drugstore, grocery store, or discount department store, then switch to a high-quality option. If you don't have a good mom-

and-pop local health food store in your area, then go to the Vitamin Shoppes website to see the brands they sell. You can then either purchase from them or buy these brands at your favorite online outlet.

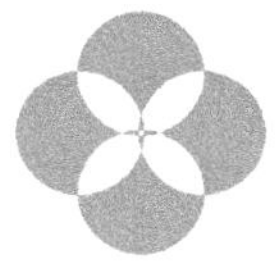

SECTION 4

Outside Help: Those Who Can Walk Alongside You, and The Tools Available to You!

Where do you go from here? If you have made a commitment to taking control of your health using natural approaches the wholistic way, then you may want to set out to build your own team of natural health care providers. Start by finding a professional person (or two) to help you along the way from time to time. When I first started my own business, I needed a team of players to help me. I found a banker, an accountant, and a lawyer. If you were to set out to build a house you would start by building your team of players including an electrician, plumber, carpenter, roofer, and others. Managing your health should be the same way. In this Section I will share with you some of the team players that could be available to you to help manage your health.

Your Team Players could also have specialty tools and testing that they might recommend or utilize in helping you restore your body back to good health. Also in this Section I'll bring some clarity on just what "supplements" are, how they can be a benefit, and how to choose quality over mass produced. And I'll also share with you some specialty testing that isn't commonly found in a conventional medicine office, as well as the proper way to interpret them.

But first, let me share with you a personal story of what this looked like for me.

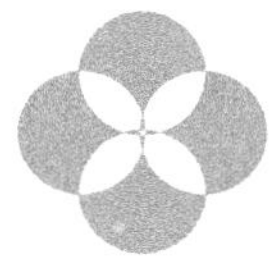

CHAPTER 10

The Truth about Natural Healthcare Practitioners: Building Your Healthcare Team

"Just as each one of you has received a special gift [a spiritual talent, an ability graciously given by God], employ it in serving one another as [is appropriate for] good stewards of God's multi-faceted grace [faithfully using the diverse, varied gifts and abilities granted to Christians by God's unmerited favor]".

—1 Peter 4:10 AMP

When I was living in Charleston, I was out jogging very early one morning before the hot sun came up. I decided to take a route through my neighborhood that I didn't normally go. I barely was out for 5 minutes when I found myself jogging on the uneven sidewalk that had been torn up a bit from construction at the elementary school. Because it was still dark, I did not see the steel chain link fence post lying across the sidewalk, still affixed to its cement base. Needless to say, that post didn't budge an inch as it caught my foot, and I went sailing arms out in front of me. I jarred my shoulder so badly I thought for sure I had dislocated it. My knees and elbows were all skinned up from the cement gravel that was all over the sidewalk; I was a mess. Fortunately, I didn't hit my head; unfortunately, it was so early in the morning that no one was out yet to see me fall and come to my rescue. I gingerly sat myself up to assess if anything was dislocated or broken—neither seemed to be the case, so I then stood up. I was crying and in horrific pain, especially in my shoulder which I couldn't seem to lift at all. I started the short trek back home and my jog was officially over for the day.

There was a little cinder block church that sat across from the entrance to the development where I was living. It had a simple wooden cross affixed to the front of the building. I felt led to walk over and just lay my shoulder against that cross and I cried out to Jesus for help and healing (spiritual health). I then proceeded the rest of the way home. The walk back gave me a little time to consider how this injury would alter my day and where I could go for additional help. I knew one thing: I did not want, nor did I have the money to go to the emergency room (I had a $5,000 insurance deductible at the time with nothing paid toward it). Plan B? I already had a meeting scheduled with another chiropractor that morning for some business, so, rather than canceling the meeting, I met her, and she adjusted me. I also called an acupuncturist I was under care with at the time to get treatment from her as well.

Before leaving for my meeting with the chiropractor, I sent an email request out to a bunch of praying friends asking for prayer for God to heal me. I also used some natural products I had in my emergency kit at home to tend to my wounds. Fortunately, I only had a few patient appointments scheduled that day and for each of them I was able to use my hand-held adjusting instrument, so that problem was solved. Two of those patients were pastors and of course prayer warriors—imagine that! I also scheduled an appointment with my massage therapist for a couple days later. Thankfully, I had a team of natural health care practitioners already in place so when the situation presented itself, all I had to do was call. And truthfully, by managing this acute injury from a wholistic approach, I was able to raise my arm up to about a 160-degree angle by the next day and the pain subsided quite quickly—God is good!

Before we delve into the various disciplines and practitioners you may want on your team, let me offer a word of caution. As a Christian, I believe that the God of the Bible is the ultimate Healer and He—and He alone—is the One who works through humans here on this earth. He is the One who has empowered and gifted every one of us to utilize the tools He has given us to bring healing to His children.

The natural health world has a tendency to draw healers from all kinds of New Age religions. Some of these practitioners believe *they* are the miracle workers, and that it is *their* "magical" energy that is doing the healing. This is witchcraft; stay as far away from this as possible—I don't care what kind of results they claim to have. I encourage you to pray about every single practitioner you choose to render care to you before you go to them. Take a look at their websites, read their bios, and learn their hobbies and interests as well as the techniques and tools they use. Of course, personal references from Godly believers in Jesus Christ who have good discernment are your best source for recommendations. All of this information can give you tremendous insight into the intent of any practitioner. I'm not saying they necessarily have to be a believer in the God of the Bible, you just don't want to go to someone who thinks *they* are the all-powerful one.

Having said this, there are also a tremendous number of wonderful natural health care practitioners who simply want to utilize the gifts, talents, and skills God has blessed them with to help you restore your body back to good health—and they would be happy to give the God of the Bible all the praise, honor, and glory for your healing!

Chiropractor

Of course, one of my favorite go-to players is a chiropractor. As we talked about earlier, chiropractors come in all various aspects of how we practice and the tools we use. First of all, I suggest looking for someone who is compassionate about you as a person and your health, someone who is willing to spend time with you, and look at your health as a whole. It's not only about how many things they can do to get you out of pain—it's the knowledge and skills they have to address your health. Most importantly, make sure they are in line with *your* health objectives. I personally prefer to use a chiropractor who can adjust my spine as well as function in the capacity as my primary care doctor. Such a practitioner will order blood work and other lab tests, spend time with me looking at my diet, and be there with their expertise should an acute situation arise whether structurally or functionally. This doctor would know when and to whom to refer me when the work is beyond their expertise. At times, the availability of a doctor who does both may not be practical. For example, where I am living now, the chiropractor I see to check my spine every 2 weeks is not a functional medicine doctor—but she is a *great* chiropractor. The functional medicine doctor who is also a chiropractor I have chosen to go to is 90 minutes away—and he is a *great* functional medicine doc. I'm sure he is a great chiropractor too, however it's just not practical for me to drive 1.5 hours one way every 2 weeks for an adjustment when another great chiropractor is just 15 minutes away. You need to set up the best team that works for you.

Acupuncturist

An acupuncturist is another great professional who can help you with your health. This is a definition from the Mayo Clinic that I found, and seems to do a good job of describing what an acupuncturist does:

> *"Traditional Chinese medicine explains acupuncture as a technique for balancing the flow of energy or life force—known as chi or qi (chee)—believed to flow through pathways (meridians) in your body. By inserting needles into specific points along these meridians, acupuncture practitioners believe that your energy flow will rebalance.*
>
> *In contrast, many Western practitioners view the acupuncture points as places to stimulate nerves, muscles, and connective tissue. Some believe that this stimulation boosts your body's natural painkillers."*

I have been to an acupuncturist who rebalanced the meridian points or energy fields in my body as well as treated me when I had an injury to my shoulder from the fall. It can be a great complement to the care you might be receiving from a functional medicine doctor, or they may be able to fulfill that role as well. Acupuncture has been around for thousands of years and has tremendous science and validity behind it—and it doesn't hurt! I have met acupuncturists who also order lab work, do nutritional consulting, prescribe supplementation, and once again look at your health as a whole.

Naturopath

A naturopath is a doctor of natural medicine. The following description of what they are trained to do comes from the American Association of Naturopathic Physicians website:

> *"Naturopathic practice includes the following diagnostic and therapeutic modalities: clinical and laboratory diagnostic testing, nutritional medicine, botanical medicine, naturopathic physical medicine (including naturopathic manipulative therapy), public health measures, hygiene, counseling, minor surgery, homeopathy, acupuncture, prescription medication, intravenous and injection therapy, and naturopathic obstetrics (natural childbirth)."*

This is who I would personally love to have as my primary care physician, provided they maintain a true wholistic natural approach, along with a chiropractor to render adjustments to remove nerve interference. A word of caution: sometimes I see and hear of naturopaths having more of a bent toward conventional medicine for some reason. I'm not sure why this is—perhaps it has something to do with where they are schooled. Unfortunately, not all states recognize naturopathic licensure, which to me is just plain wrong. My theory is this may be the reason some practice under a medical doctor's license and are therefore obligated to stay more on the medical course.

Nutritionist

A nutritionist is another player that could be beneficial to have on your team, especially if you don't have a functional medicine doc on your team—this might be all you need. They also look at you as a whole person and determine the right foods for you and your body, as an individual. Remember, a true nutritionist doesn't count calories; they look at the nutrients that might be depleted and recommend the foods best for you. Depending on the state and any other licenses that they may hold, they may be able to order blood work and/or specialty lab testing like hormone tests, hidden food sensitivities, etc. They may also utilize tools like other natural health care professionals to determine your vitamin and mineral deficiencies and those that can help rebalance the body.

NOTE: I know we covered this earlier, but I believe it bears repeating—there is a big difference between a nutritionist and a dietician. A dietician is trained and licensed under the conventional medical board and their philosophy is to manage the disease. They have also recently changed the name of their association from the American Dieticians Association (ADA) to the Academy of Nutrition and Dietetics (AND), which in my opinion is a bit deceiving—their objectives are very different from those of a true nutritionist. The information you find on the internet will be dominated by dieticians, so beware. Look to see who they are licensed under and go from there.

What is a Hydro Therapist?

I'm all about logistics, especially when I set out to do something new. For a long time, I read about and heard people suggesting incorporating colonics into my health regimen. As you now know,

I am definitely a firm believer that the digestive system is a vital system to the health of anyone's body, and it needs to be well taken care of, but I just could never seem to get past the logistics of doing enemas on myself. I would hear instructions that would say things like "get in the bathtub…" The bathtub? Is that with or without water in the tub?! Really, I asked myself that! I just couldn't picture it, and I also wondered why the bathtub was used. I'm still not sure of the answer to this…

Fortunately, I have several *good* friends and colleagues who ventured these paths before me that I felt comfortable asking them. They were kind and patient enough to explain the logistics to me, but I'm not here to share that with you today. You can search the internet if you really want to know!

My personal recommendation, however, is if you want—or even more importantly need—a thorough cleansing of the colon, go to a professional hydro therapist as I eventually did. Unfortunately, if you live in a smaller town, and especially a town where folks aren't strong supporters of taking care of their health, you might have to travel to a larger town to find one—but it's worth it.

A hydro therapist is also trained and licensed. Cleanliness is vital to their profession, as is a gentle bedside manner—both literally and emotionally. I have been to two different hydro therapists and they both were nothing less than the utmost professionals. The benefit of utilizing the services of a professional hydro therapist is that their equipment can cleanse the entire length of the colon. When using a home enema/colonic, at best you are just getting beyond the very last portion of the colon called the sigmoid colon. Some people who do their own say it gets further up the colon than that, but I have my doubts. The length of the entire colon, including two major bends, is approximately 5 feet long. Unless you are inserting a tube that is at least close to that length, or one with a powerful water source that has enough pressure to reach the other end, I don't believe you are getting a sufficient cleansing.

Whether you are doing a home treatment or utilizing a professional, you want to absolutely be certain to supplement your nutritional intake with a good probiotic, as again in my opinion, you are pulling out the good bacteria along with anything else that might have been stagnant in there.

Picture a dirty, fairly empty, casserole dish with baked-on food; it needs some soaking and scrubbing in order for it to become fully clean. That's how your colon can get if it is not routinely completely emptied after each meal. Most people do not experience this. With 70 percent of our immune system in our digestive system, a clean colon is vital to our health.

Massage Therapist

Massage therapy is the manipulation of the body's soft tissues, such as muscles, tendons, ligaments, and skin, by using various degrees of pressure and movement. It is typically performed by a licensed professional called a massage therapist and it's often used as a treatment for various medical conditions. Some of the classic benefits of massage therapy are:

- reduced muscle and joint pain and tension.
- reduced stress levels.
- improved immune system function.
- it can induce a state of relaxation.

Having a massage can be another one of those natural techniques that a person might have to wrap their minds around before receiving its benefits. Some women in particular are more modest than others. They, and even some men, may have been abused in their lives, especially as a child, so there is tremendous discomfort about disrobing for a stranger, let alone allowing them to put their hands on your naked or near-naked body. There can also be other inhibitions about doing so. For some men and women, it comes down to the comfort level of whether they want a man or a woman therapist touching them. This is a discipline, like colonics, that requires an extreme amount of trust in the professional rendering the care.

To be honest, I don't really recall when I received my first massage, or whether it was from a man or a woman. I do recall receiving a massage from a friend of mine who was in massage therapy school. If you wanted to overcome your shyness about receiving a massage, this school would do it for you! It literally was one great big room, and each massage therapist had their own workstation. You would disrobe (to whatever degree you were comfortable) with just the privacy of a sheet held up for you! Talk about intimidation! Do not fear—this is NOT the norm for massage therapists rendering professional private care to you, where you will disrobe in private and to the level of your personal comfort.

The benefits of a medical or therapeutic massage are tremendous. As a chiropractic physician, I had a massage therapist in my office whose work would complement the chiropractic adjustments. My chiropractor today has the same. A massage therapist is uniquely trained to relax and loosen the muscles, as well as to work out toxins that get stored in the muscles. Once the muscles are relaxed, the chiropractor can render their care, allowing the bones to move back into their proper alignment more easily and stay there longer. Each discipline is a tremendous complement to the other.

Of course, there are all types of massages; here are a few types and techniques used:

- Swedish
- Aromatherapy
- Deep Tissue
- Trigger
- Medical
- Shiatsu
- Sports
- Hot Stone
- Reflexology

You can learn more about the benefits of massage and the different types by going to their professional website: www.amtamassage.org.

Thermography

The last natural treatment tool I will share with you, and one that most people are not aware of, is thermography.

Thermography is a high-tech health screening tool (a high-definition infrared camera) that creates a digital map of your body and temperature patterns, which may show abnormalities indicative of inflammation (or abnormal heat spots on the body).

Thermography is most commonly used as a safer alternative for women instead of a mammogram. Thermography will detect hyper-cellular activity, through the visualization of temperature patterns, long before irregular tissue activity would ever be detected on a mammogram. It is noninvasive. In fact, the woman's body is never touched by either the practitioner or any equipment. The detection of hyper-cellular activity is *not* affirmative for cancer; it signifies something is going on beneath the surface. Should there be an indication of hyper-cellular activity, you could then pursue further studies to rule out any pathologies. On the flip side, having a mammogram uses radiation, which is known to cause cancer. It's also very uncomfortable as most women know and men might only imagine.

The service I use is actually under the supervision of a medical doctor who has a technician travel with a mobile unit. The technician just needs a small office or room that provides privacy to do their work. The first time I became aware of this tool and service was when I worked at the health food store. The technician would provide us with her schedule a month or so out, and customers would schedule appointments with her in advance. In addition to health food stores, she also would visit compounding pharmacies and practitioner's offices. The medical doc is the one who reads the reports and emails them to the patients. Simple as that. It is also very inexpensive—probably somewhere between \$100–\$150 depending on the area. You can also have other parts of your body scanned or even a full body scan.

I highly recommend this service and going this route over a mammogram.

Your Wellness Team, in Summary

These descriptions are very general, and the practitioners are each unique in what they may or may not offer. They also will vary from state to state as to what they may or may not legally be able to do. For example, chiropractors are the only complementary and alternative practitioners that are licensed in all 50 states. A lot of the time one practitioner may hold several different licenses like an acupuncturist might have a nutrition degree as well, or a chiropractor may also be able to do acupuncture. You may even find some medical doctors (MDs) who have "seen the light" and now practice fully as a true functional medicine practitioner. I love these folks because they have literally experienced both sides of the fence. Personally, I think the more diverse a practitioner is, the better. It shows me they truly desire to approach the person wholistically and want to utilize as many tools as possible to do so.

The best thing to do is research the practitioner(s) you are considering. Look at their websites, ask others in your community what they have heard about them, ask for references from the practitioner you are considering using, and interview that practitioner. You may also want to have several professionals helping you. You could ask an existing practitioner to make a recommendation for another in an area that they don't cover. If that is the case, however, make sure that they are communicating with each other; you should not be the messenger between them. It is more important than anything that you trust the person or people on your Wellness Team.

Once you are able to trust them with your health, you need to let them do their job and follow their recommendations. They know what they are doing, or you wouldn't trust them. You are a unique individual and no one person should be treated exactly like the next. It took your body a long time to get to the place of disease or imbalance that it is, so it is going to take some time to restore that body back to good health. Give your practitioner, or team of practitioners, time to do their work. Above all, don't have "Dr. Internet" as one of your wellness team members!

A closing word of caution: There are many, many styles of practicing out there in all of these "alternative" and natural arenas. The world of natural medicine has a tendency to draw what I would call "new age" practitioners. I know from personal experience that some of them are operating from a place of ego, thinking it is their own superpower that is causing the healing, and at times even with other "spirits." I know this might sound far-fetched, but it is happening nonetheless. I caution you to be careful who is "laying hands" on you. There are some techniques and practitioners that claim to be doing "energy work" and their work entails "their energy influencing your energy." This is witchcraft. God alone is the only One who heals—we are simply His vessels He works through.

But don't let a few practitioners in any one of these natural fields distort your view of the majority. When someone asks me what I think of a particular discipline or practitioner I always ask, "what is the intent of the practitioner?" That's why I personally prefer to work with a Christian first (and even then, assess their intent) or someone who carries themself with the utmost professionalism and is not relying on their own spirit to do the work that only God, through them, can do.

Call to Action: Start building your Wholistic Wellness Team. Make a list of who you might already have on your team, even if you have only seen them once. If you like and trust them, keep them on your list and build your team from there.

Even if you don't feel you need specific services at the moment, start researching them now. That way, if a time comes when you need them quickly, you won't be making decisions from a place of panic.

You could even go as far as scheduling a consultation appointment with them just to get established and interview them. Maybe they looked good on their website, but once you met them in person, they did not resonate with you.

Above all, pray about establishing a relationship with each one. Ask God who He wants to be rendering care to the body He created.

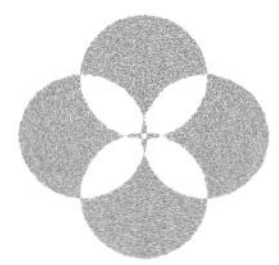

CHAPTER 11

The Truth About Supplements

So God said, "Behold, I have given you every plant yielding seed that is on the surface of the entire earth, and every tree which has fruit yielding seed; it shall be food for you;"

—Genesis 1:29 AMP

Hopefully you are beginning to realize by now that a lot of the barriers to our health lie in the way we think about health. Much of our wrong thinking comes from years of being told one thing, when in fact the total opposite is true. No wonder people get frustrated with achieving good health and simply give up. Revealing these truths drives me and I hope it helps you, so much so that it gives you an "aha moment" and the light bulb of hope goes on in your heart!

Let's next explore the world of natural supplements, and I'll start off by defining what I mean by "supplement." Technically, a better phrase is "dietary supplement." According to the Dietary Supplement Health and Education Act (DSHEA) of 1994 the definition of a dietary supplement is as follows:

> *"A dietary supplement is a product taken by mouth that contains a "dietary ingredient" intended to supplement the diet. The 'dietary ingredients' in these products may include: vitamins, minerals, herbs or other botanicals, amino acids, and substances such as enzymes, organ tissues, glandulars, and metabolites. Dietary supplements can also be extracts or concentrates, and may be found in many forms such as tablets, capsules, softgels, gelcaps, liquids, or powders."*

The key words here are "supplement the diet." Our health should always start with food first.

Quality Supplements versus Cheap Synthetics

I want to next address the difference between quality whole food-based supplements versus cheap synthetics.

Before we delve in, let me remind you and I repeat this with all seriousness—your health and your life are no place to pinch pennies. Way too often, our health and the means to obtain it and keep it are put far too low on the priority list of our time and our finances. People will splurge on high-end technology, homes, cars, and vacations and all the luxuries that go along with these things but will say they can't afford to take care of their health. Remember, YOU are valuable! YOU have a divine purpose and reason for being here on this earth. So please, please don't cut corners when it comes to your health. Now onto synthetic vs. whole food-based supplements.

First of all, synthetic supplements are made from manufactured chemicals that might resemble real food chemically under a microscope, but do not function as real food in your body. Depending on where you buy them and what brand you are buying, they could very well have a bunch of unhealthy additives in them, including toxic metals like lead. This is truly counterproductive to your health. You will not find quality whole food-based supplements in the mass-market stores like discount department stores, grocery stores, chain drug stores, or dollar stores.

When you consume synthetic Vitamin C for example, the body has to look for all the other vitamins and minerals it needs first, in order to do the work that Vitamin C does. No vitamin or mineral found in nature functions independently of other vitamins and minerals—they all need each other in order to function properly, as they are designed to do. Studies have shown that excessive Vitamin C could be harmful to you. However, these studies have been done using synthetic Vitamin C and that *could* be harmful to you. First of all, anything synthetic—food, supplements, pharmaceuticals, skin care products, etc., are foreign substances to the body and cause a burden on the liver to get rid of them. Second, it's robbing the body of the other vitamins and minerals it needs in order to semi-function as real Vitamin C.

The problem with cheap retail products, like those supplements discussed above, is they are mass produced and therefore lack the true efficacy needed to really be beneficial. In fact, they can actually be harmful when laden with pesticides, herbicides, and even heavy metals. They can say an ingredient is in their product, when in essence a trace amount of it is in there (or none at all) and they have told the "truth." Vitamin C is an excellent example of this. There can be a minute trace of what was once Vitamin C, but by the time it has all been processed, it is nothing like true Vitamin C. In fact, this is what is known as a "synthetic" supplement. Echinacea, which is an herb, is another example. Herbs have many parts that can be used for healing—the flower, stem, seeds, leaves, roots, etc., and each of these parts serves a different purpose (or none at all). Some are more readily available than others, so the cheaper more available parts are quite often used in place of the effective part. The *root* of the echinacea plant is what is valuable to support the immune system, however less expensive parts of the plant are quite often used instead and labeled "echinacea"—which in reality it is, but not effective for the purpose we were taking it for.

The same goes for the packaged, processed, and manufactured foods that are "fortified" with vitamins and minerals. The natural vitamins and minerals that may have been there at the beginning stages of production have been killed off through the manufacturing process, so these food-like substances are fortified with synthetic vitamins and/or minerals making you think that you are getting more than you would if you ate real food. In fact, this is contrary to the truth!

Whole food-based supplements are a far better choice, and actual whole food supplements (those made literally from real foods) are the best choice. You will most likely find your whole food-based supplements and whole food supplements in your independent health food stores, and places like Earth Fare, Whole Foods, or Trader Joe's. Vitamin Shoppe seems to have quality brands as well. These are all going to be much more conscious of the quality of their products because that's what they are known for, and their reputation is on the line otherwise. The majority, if not all, of the supplement companies these stores carry are members of the Natural Products Association. In order to be a member of the Association, they have to subject their products to third-party verification. This means an unbiased laboratory, not affiliated with any supplement company, tests the products for purity as well as the truth of their labeling—meaning what they say is in there truly is. If you have questions on the efficacy of any brand, consider them through these filters first.

For the most part, the professional grade (nutraceutical) supplements and *quality* retail are very conscientious about quality control, clean ingredients, minimal fillers, proper quantities, and correct ingredients in their products. They are also very conscious of the peak harvesting time for the herbs and other ingredients that might be used to formulate their products.

As might be expected, the price of quality supplements that are actually going to perform as expected is going to be higher. Spending just a few dollars less on something that isn't going to do what it is supposed to, and in fact could be detrimental to your health is, in my opinion, costlier; you've thrown your money away and probably *caused* health problems (at least if used over a longer period of time).

There is also controversy about natural supplements not being regulated by the US Food and Drug Administration (F.D.A.). There definitely are pluses and minuses to this. If they *were* truly regulated, the only way you would have access to them would be through a medical doctor via prescription, which in essence would be controlled by the drug companies. Because they are *not* regulated, there is no oversight of what a manufacturer says is in there and whether it actually is.

Multi-level marketing products are also a concern for me. This is not because the product itself is not any good; rather it is because of the messages they send. In fact, I myself have used and prescribed some multi-level products. Too often these products are touted as the "miracle cure." Here is an example: I was talking with a childhood friend on the phone one day; we hadn't talked in the last 30 years but thanks to the advent of Facebook we connected once again. We got talking about health (as is usually the case if you end up in a conversation with me for any length of time), and she said "I can't believe I'm getting ready to tell you about this, but..." She proceeded to tell me about all the fantastic properties of this particular multi-level marketing product (of course she did not reveal to me it was multi-level marketing). Before she said the name of the product I said, "let me guess, it's _____." And she said "no, it's ______!" My point is, the sales pitch was exactly the same as another product that was the latest trend at the time, but a different product! They all seem to pitch the same "miracle cure" message.

Multi-level marketing supplements lead to that wrong thinking of "outward, inward." Here is my symptom, give me something just to make me "feel" better, and in this case it's the latest "miracle cure." The multi-level marketing products always seem to promote how much "energy" you have with them. Now I know I am generalizing here, but my question still remains focused on the root cause of your symptoms. Folks, don't just mask your symptoms—even with a natural product—get to the root cause of the problem first.

A word of caution here: just because taking something makes you "feel" good doesn't necessarily mean it is benefiting your health. Alcohol or cocaine may make someone "feel" good (at least in the short term), but they certainly are not beneficial to their health. The way to tell if your supplements are working is through reassessments of your health using the measuring sticks that prompted you to supplement in the first place—things like lab testing etc.—and not just because an article in a magazine said "if you have these symptoms, take this." Assess if your overall health is improving as a result of taking care of it—not just by taking a "magic pill" but by making comprehensive lifestyle changes for the better. Don't expect changes by taking a pill and doing nothing else to help yourself. You will be setting yourself up for disappointment, if not wasting your money on the supplements. By all means, don't pinch pennies when it comes to your health; make your health a priority and purchase quality supplements to support your health plan.

To repeat an important point from the first chapter—there are some supplements that I believe we all need, ongoing, no matter how healthy we are. Even with the best of diets, we still aren't getting the full nutrients we need from our food any longer. By eating foods on the "Short List of Acidic/Inflammatory Foods" such as fast food, fried food, packaged and processed foods, and sugars, we are not just missing the nutrients we need, but these food-like substances are actually robbing the body of the nutrients it does have. Here are the foundational supplements I feel we all need:

- Probiotic
- Full-spectrum digestive enzyme
- Possibly hydrochloric acid (most people need this)
- Multi-vitamin and mineral
- Essential Fatty Acids (EFAs), e.g., Omega 3s, Fish Oil, etc.
- Vitamin D
- Magnesium (ideally a transdermal one; I like the one made by Mg12)

These are the very basics. A lot of people need others as well—like CoQ10 for cardiovascular health in particular. All cells in the body need CoQ10; it is important for our immune function. Also, any kind of cholesterol medications you may be taking will rob the body of CoQ10, so you will want to supplement this vital nutrient back into the body. Every cell in the body also needs iodine; the thyroid, breast tissue, uterus, ovaries, and testicles especially utilize a heavy saturation of iodine. Chlorine and fluoride typically found in our tap water and bromide usually found in baked goods will rob your body of iodine. We will talk more about that below.

If you are also trying to restore the body back to good health, you could use more specific supplements to help assist in the healing process for whatever area is out of balance. Some supplements should be taken in an ongoing manner as part of your lifetime health regimen; others should only be taken until you have reached the health results you set out to achieve.

Supplements collectively cover a broad spectrum of subcategories. Let's move on to explaining these subcategories by breaking them down a little further.

What are Vitamins?

The word vitamin is just one component that makes up supplements. A lot of people will ask for a vitamin, when in fact they may be wanting an herb, or a digestive enzyme, or a multitude of other things. So, know what you really want; otherwise, you may be led to something you didn't really want or need. There are two basic categories of vitamins: fat soluble and water soluble.

Fat-soluble Vitamins

Vitamins that can be stored in our human body are called fat-soluble vitamins. Vitamins A, D, E, and K are fat soluble vitamins, which dissolve in fat and are stored in liver and fat tissues until they are needed. Fat-soluble vitamins cannot be easily excreted from the body except vitamin K, so they are toxic if taken in excessive amounts. Absorption of these vitamins totally depends upon efficient fat intake and absorption. In healthy individuals, eating a normal and healthy diet will not lead to toxicity of these vitamins. Vitamin A (also known as retinol) helps eyes adjust to changes in light. It also plays a role in bone growth, reproduction, regulation of the immune system, and cell division. Vitamin D can be obtained through sunlight and helps in absorption of calcium from the small intestine which then is absorbed into our bones and makes them stronger. In children, vitamin D is essential for the development of stronger bones and healthy teeth. Vitamin E acts as an antioxidant which protects vitamins A and C, red blood cells, and essential fatty acids from destruction. Vitamin K is produced by bacteria that are present in our gut and helps in normal blood clotting, production of proteins for blood, bones, and kidneys, and promotes bone health.

Water-soluble Vitamins

Those vitamins which cannot be stored in our body are called water-soluble vitamins. Vitamin B-complex and vitamin C are water-soluble vitamins which are dissolved in water and eliminated in urine. We require a continuous daily supplement of these vitamins in our diet. Vitamin B-complexes are divided into eight groups. Vitamin B1, or thiamine, is important for maintaining our nervous system; it also helps to release energy from food and promotes normal appetite.

Vitamin B2, or riboflavin, promotes good vision and healthy skin. Vitamin B3, or niacin, helps with normal enzyme function, promotes healthy skin and nerves, and normal appetite. Pantothenic acid (B5) helps in the formation of hormones. Vitamin B6, or pyridoxine, aids protein metabolism and formation of red blood cells (RBCs). Folic acid also promotes RBC formation. Vitamin B12, or cobalamin, aids in the building of our genetic material. Biotin aids in metabolism of fats, protein, and carbohydrates. Lastly, vitamin C, or ascorbic acid, helps in the formation of collagen, a connective tissue that holds muscles, bones, and tissues together. It also helps with wound healing, maintaining the nervous system, and in the absorption of iron.

What are Minerals?

I told you earlier about the water ionizer and how my body was depleted in electrolytes. That is just one example of the vitalness of minerals. Electrolytes are minerals that are dissolved when mixed with water. Our bodies have vitamins, minerals, and even trace minerals. The body needs all of them in the right balance, the right quantity, the right ratio, and most importantly, the right biochemical form. I think most people have heard about sodium, potassium, and calcium. They truly are vital to life.

Women especially seem to be obsessed with having enough calcium and not knowing enough about it except that the doctor told them to take it so they don't end up with a hip fracture in the future. They go grab a bottle while they are out at the discount store picking up the pet food. Any bottle, the cheapest, because they are "all the same, right?" Wrong! Remember, there is a difference between mass produced and quality.

There is also another vital mineral, magnesium. All minerals have different biochemical forms—some are better than others and some can even be harmful. However, one of the more important, yet the most overlooked and underestimated mineral is magnesium; it is known as the "master mineral." All of the other vitamins and minerals need the sufficient quantity and the right form of magnesium in order to function as God intended.

I love magnesium so much because it is such an easy fix, and deficiency of it can lead to the root cause of so many problems. We are quite frequently, if not chronically, low in magnesium. Medications deplete the body of magnesium; stress does too. Anxiety and depression are almost always rooted in a magnesium deficiency, not "medication" deficiencies. Serotonin needs magnesium in order to be released. Melatonin needs magnesium too to help us with sleep. Calcium is the muscle contractor; magnesium is the muscle relaxer—our heart and every other muscle in the body need both. Too often the body has too much calcium and not enough magnesium; an example is leg cramps. Your colon is also a muscle. If you are constipated, you are most likely not only deficient in water but probably magnesium as well.

My favorite way to dose with magnesium is transdermal, meaning a topical oil form. If you wake in the morning and have a loose bowel movement, you've taken a little too much—just back down a bit on your dosage. I particularly like the brand Mg12. They have all kinds of magnesium products, from balms to deodorants and shampoos, to products containing arnica for sore muscles. I use MagneSport balm on the bottoms of my feet every night following a day of backpacking. Not only is my body under extreme stress from the rigorous day of backpacking but my feet are also sore, so it's a double benefit! Mg12 is a Christian company who puts a drop of frankincense and myrrh in each batch of their oils and prays over each batch. The salts come from the Dead Sea—a quality product all the way around.

For much greater information on the benefits and necessity of magnesium, please read Dr. Carolyn Dean's book *The Miracle of Magnesium*—an excellent and eye-opening read.

The Truth about Herbs

Beyond the more common terms like vitamins and minerals, I realize that the world of natural health can seem very confusing, misleading, skeptical, and even scary to a lot of people. I want to take the next few pages and share about some of the terminology, different styles of natural healing, power, and true efficacy of each; hopefully I can demystify things for you. A couple of terms I want to define are homeopathy/homeopathic and herbology/herbalist, and what they are and the benefits of each.

I have attended several Medicines of the Earth Herbal Symposiums. Every time I was blown away by what I learned and the amazing outcomes the doctors there have experienced using herbs, so that is where I would like to go next—plants and herbs.

I will be honest with you, until I attended these symposiums, I thought of herbs, herbology, and herbalists as something a little "out there"—in other words, not overly effective for health and wellness. I could not have been more wrong! Not only are they so amazing, but there is an incredible amount of *science* behind their efficacy too. These are not just Grandma's remedies for the common cold or an upset stomach, although they are good for that too; I'm talking about major things like digestive disorders, hormonal imbalances, sleep disturbances, autoimmune diseases, and yes, even cancer. The science, in a lot of cases, is cited in prominent US medical journals. I had lunch with an oncology nurse one day at one of the symposiums. She was absolutely flabbergasted that the proof of the efficacy of these plants and herbs was in their very own medical journals and yet were hardly ever acknowledged, let alone used for healing.

The first year I attended the Symposium I was totally in awe of the incredible knowledge of the presenters and healthcare practitioners that were at this conference. In comparison, I felt like I knew nothing when it came to natural healthcare, even though I had been in it for 15+ years at that time. Not only was I impressed with the knowledge of the people there, but I was amazed by what we can do with the plants and herbs that at times are practically in our own backyards—or could be. The strength and potency are incredible and a lot of times equal to or even far greater than a drug. So much so that it's the reason we want to report any herbs we are taking to our doctor before being prescribed a pharmaceutical medication. This is similar to a doctor's need to know what medications you are taking before prescribing you something else for caution of drug interaction. After all, herbs are the base of a lot of pharmaceutical drugs.

God gave us these plants to not only nourish our bodies but to heal them as well. They can be used medicinally or for cooking. They can be used in teas or be applied topically. They can be consumed fresh, cooked, dried, in tinctures and extracts, or ground down and put in a capsule. There is a lot to be said for "Grandma's secret remedy." In fact, I started having greater respect for plants and herbs even prior to the Symposium. This actually started with some of YOU! Yes, those of you who used to come into the rural health food store where I worked and bought dried herbs that I never even heard of before. You may have thought I was simply being nosey, but I was curious and wanted to learn what you were going to do with Mullein Leaf or Marshmallow Root, or a slew of other herbs that people were buying. I was learning from you—and I was astonished!

I am not an expert on herbs by any means and I'm still learning myself, but I will encourage you like I have been encouraged. Go to the library or bookstore and get a book on herbs—ideally those native to your geographical area. Pick five or ten of them and start studying and learning all the benefits of just one herb. They each can have many benefits. Start applying them and using them, perhaps even grow them—have fun with them! Make fresh tea for yourself, dry them out, and consume them. See what a difference they can make in your health. You might decide to take a course in herbology—the opportunities are endless. You might even find out that *this* could be *your* unique, divine calling here on this earth—making medicines from the tools God gave us to help heal others—now wouldn't that be awesome!?

In addition to the right foods (and keep in mind that herbs are foods too), water, exercise, sleep, and good nerve supply, the use of medicinal herbs is another tool that you can use to help bring your body back to good health and keep it there. Or better yet, use all these tools including herbs, to *prevent* all the diseases we hear about today. The best place to buy dried herbs or in supplement form would be at a good health food store. They usually have knowledgeable staff there as well as some books that can help guide you as to which herbs would fit your needs best. Herbs are quite often sold in bulk so you can purchase as little or as much as you want or need. Frontier Co-op is a great source of bulk herbs too.

Whatever you end up doing with this new knowledge on herbs, be sure *not* to underestimate the power of these natural medicines God has so generously given to us to use for our good.

The Truth about Homeopathy

I absolutely love using and recommending homeopathic remedies! You possibly have used them in the past too but may have been unaware that you were even doing so. My favorite brand is King Bio but there are also other wonderful companies as well—Heel, Boiron, and Hylands to name a few more. *These* you can find in, and it's okay to buy from, your local drug store or grocery store. Once again, I am not an expert in this field, but the majority of what I have learned about homeopathy I have learned from Dr. Frank King.

Homeopathy works on a molecular level along the energetic pathways in our body, which is the nervous system. Unlike herbs, vitamins, and minerals, homeopathics bypass the digestive system, which in a lot of cases is not functioning properly, especially in someone whose health is compromised. The energetic material in the homeopathic remedy is picked up by the sublingual nerve (located under the tongue) and goes directly into the nervous system and the quickest route to the brain. Molecular function controls the cellular function in our bodies.

Think of the energetic pathways (the nervous system) as the communication network of our bodies. When the body is compromised on even the most cellular level, the communication is disrupted in the body. You could also think of the energetic pathways similar to the fiber-optic "wires" for our cell phones; when there is disruption in the signal, we lose connection with whom we are speaking. Or think of the energetic pathways as the electrical system in our house, where we lose power if there is an interruption. In these examples, the homeopathic remedies act as the cell phone repairman or the electrician who fixes the disruption. Homeopathy "fixes" the misfiring of nerve signals in our bodies.

The reason I love using homeopathic remedies is because (according to the government) homeopathy is the only natural remedy that is allowed to claim to "cure." Although, in my humble opinion, real food and herbs can cure too, the government says otherwise (but that is a discussion for another day!). There are no side effects or drug interactions using homeopathic remedies. It is absolutely safe for a person on 20 medications to use homeopathic remedies; a day-old infant can be given a homeopathic remedy. According to Dr. King, one can use up to 4 different remedies at the same time and still be effective. After that, the body starts getting confused and cannot process the bioenergetic information optimally. You may be wondering what happens if you try a remedy and it's not the right one for you and your body. The answer is nothing; the worst that can happen is nothing, meaning the area that is out of balance simply won't heal. There is a good likelihood you need the remedy somewhere in your body, even if you are not "feeling" it, so it still would not be a waste.

So, what is in a homeopathic remedy? Dr. Samuel Hahnemann founded the science of homeopathy in the late 1700s. Through numerous experiments, he advanced the theory that "likes are cured by likes," establishing what has become a verified law of pharmacology, the *Law of Similars*. Vaccinations are made under this same premise of "like cures like." The ingredients can be a formula of anything from plants, herbs, vitamins, minerals, and/or animal glandulars.

I am going to give you a very basic description of how a homeopathic remedy is made from these ingredients (I hope I am not doing Dr. King or homeopathy a disservice by my simplified explanation!).

Water has the ability to hold the "memory" of the molecular pattern of any ingredient(s). The formulation of ingredients is boiled in a vat of water (in some cases, a very high-energetic pure water), then the water is poured off and reserved. A potentiation process, which increases the energy of the formula and gives the strength and effectiveness of the remedy, is applied to the water. Some brands then put the water into a tablet or pellet form, to dissolve it under the tongue.

I know this all might sound a little confusing, and some might find it hard to believe that something so simple can really be effective, especially for serious health problems. But using homeopathic remedies along with lifestyle changes such as diet, sleep, exercise, water, and good spinal hygiene can yield amazing results!

Personally, I found it hard to believe I could push a few buttons on a little rectangular hand-held device without any wires attached to it and speak to my mom in California. I can't see it working, I can't taste it working, I can't feel it working but I can hear it working. Homeopathic remedies work the same way; you might not be able to see, hear, or even taste it (they are tasteless), but you will be able to feel them working. Give them a try—it won't hurt you and it can only do good. I think you will be pleasantly surprised and come to love them like I do.

The Truth about Mushrooms!

There is one more type of supplement I love that I don't want to overlook: mycelium or fungi, i.e., *legal* mushrooms. I am not talking about hallucinogenic mushrooms but rather medicinal mushrooms such as Reishi, Maitake, Chaga, Lions Mane, and Cordyceps as well as a combination of these mushrooms. They have tremendous healing properties, especially for the immune system and can even address conditions like cancer. You should do some research and make sure, like every other supplement, that they are quality. One company, but certainly not the only one, is Host Defense. To learn more about the efficacy of the healing properties of mushrooms, and even how to harvest them yourself, I suggest Paul Stamet's book *Mycelium Running, How Mushrooms Can Help Save the World.*

Call to Action: I encourage you to learn more about these natural products that are not as common to you like herbal medicine, homeopathy, and mushrooms. Most likely these are a little foreign to you (especially the last two), but they have tremendous healing abilities. If you are not confident in what they can do or how they work, you will probably have a tendency to avoid them.

By understanding how they work and what they can do, you will be able to expand the "tools in your wellness toolbox" and utilize them when needed with confidence!

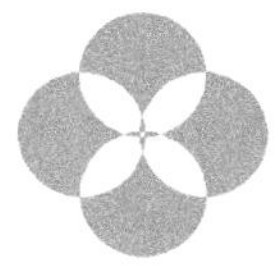

CHAPTER 12

The Truth About Wholistic Health Tests

"But test all things carefully [so you can recognize what is good]. Hold firmly to that which is good."

—1 Thessalonians 5:21 AMP

When I first started taking my post-doctorate courses in internal disorders, I quickly became amazed at how many different tests that conventional medicine simply does not utilize—and I continue to learn of more.

Every once in a while, even the doctor has to go beyond the old adage "doctor heal thyself," and reach out to colleagues for help. That's what I had to do recently. As a result of getting COVID-19, a manufactured toxin, the Epstein Barr virus which I had acquired as a child became reactivated, causing inflammation and triggering some autoimmune responses to the smooth muscles in my body.

It required a lot of "doctor detective work" to come to that conclusion. In fact, it truly took several months before we got to the bottom of what was going on. High blood pressure initially sent me to my doctor's office. I just couldn't seem to get the blood pressure down by doctoring myself. I decided to reach out to a practitioner who was like-minded and on the same page as me in pursuing my objective of getting to the root *cause* of the problem and restoring my body to good health using natural approaches. He utilized all kinds of specialty lab tests I had never heard of, even beyond what I am sharing with you here. Had I gone to a conventional medical doctor's office complaining of high blood pressure, I would undoubtedly be on medication the rest of my life 10 minutes after I arrived. Problem solved? Not.

Let's move on to the differences between the way traditional medicine and natural medicine practitioners interpret some blood markers as well as the other tools used to analyze your health that traditional medicine typically does not use.

There are two main differences between how conventional medicine and functional medicine docs order and interpret lab work. First, conventional medicine almost always orders very limited lab tests. They seem to order labs that would confirm their preconceived diagnosis, because insurance companies require the physician to submit their requests for lab work with a diagnosis code. This never made sense to me as a functional medicine practitioner—I needed lab work to help me determine the diagnosis, not confirm my guess of what I *think* is going on. Functional medicine doctors will typically order much more comprehensive panels for initial intake. We want to see how each of these markers are affecting the others. I commonly see incomplete thyroid panels ordered. More on that in a minute.

The second difference is, once the conventional medicine doctor receives the results for the limited lab work they ordered, they simply look to see if something is high or something is low. If nothing is out of the "normal" reference range, they dub you "healthy," i.e., "nothing" is wrong. This is the report I hear over and over again from people who bring me their lab results. They tell me "everything is good, my doctor said my labs look great," yet they are standing there in front of me feeling lousy. This goes back to that spectrum of health we talked about earlier—just because your lab work doesn't fall within the diseased range doesn't mean you are "healthy."

We are all somewhere on the spectrum of health; we might not be diseased, but we always have room for improvement because none of us is 100 percent healthy. Most likely, if a marker is high, they may prescribe you medication for it. For example, if glucose is high just one time—bam—you are dubbed diabetic and given that prescription for a medicine quicker than you can say "chocolate bar!"

Functional medicine practitioners look beyond the given reference range, which varies from laboratory to laboratory, region by region of the country. We will see a lot more "highs" and "lows" in our interpretations—meaning you are not necessarily diseased, but something is going on sub-clinically. We also take all the lab markers and their results and analyze them comprehensively, not just what is high or low. There also seems to be a trend for conventional medicine to focus more on labs when they are too high as opposed to too low. Let's take a closer look at the right way to interpret cholesterol—the truth.

The Truth about Cholesterol

There are basically five markers in a cholesterol panel: total cholesterol, HDL (the so-called good cholesterol), LDL (the so-called bad one), VLDL (very low-density lipoprotein), triglycerides, and the coronary risk factor (CRF, otherwise shown on lab reports as HDL:Total ratio).

If we are looking at the cholesterol panel from a coronary/cardiovascular risk concern, then it should stand to reason that the most important number on this panel should be the CRF or HDL:Total ratio. Most of the time people aren't even aware of this number. Often, it's the "Total" and the "LDL" that are the focus, because this is what the drug companies have drilled into the medical doctors and patients alike. We have all heard that if our cholesterol is over 200, we have high cholesterol and need to be on medications so we won't have a heart attack and die. There is such a fear factor placed on people that if they don't take drugs and do what the medical doctor tells them, they will surely die. While this may be true if your objective is to manage your disease, this is not your only option! In my opinion, the better option is to take control of your health and restore your body using natural approaches.

When traditional medicine looks at your cholesterol numbers, it is to see if you are at RISK for heart disease. If that's true, then it would make sense the most important number on the cholesterol blood panel *should* be the CRF (Coronary *Risk* Factor). However, that number is rarely discussed. Everyone seems to know what their total cholesterol is (at least if they have had it checked), but they never seem to know what their CRF is. This is because the drug companies use the *total* cholesterol number as their marketing tool.

More recently, it was even said *everyone* should be on cholesterol medications, including kids, simply for prevention. Really?

I would like to take a moment and just point out a few things to you. First, the so-called "high" cholesterol is not a disease; it's just one risk factor. Others include obesity, smoking, high blood pressure, diabetes, and family history of heart disease to name a few.

Second, our bodies absolutely need cholesterol. All of our hormones are made up of cholesterol, and we must have our hormones functioning properly in order for our bodies to function properly. In contrast, natural medicine considers a total cholesterol number below 140 a possible ominous sign. This could mean that something major is happening in your body and you might not even be aware of it—fatty congested liver, cancer, and any number of other degenerative diseases—and using medications forces the number lower. Cholesterol medications also lower both the LDL ("bad" cholesterol) *and* the HDL ("good" cholesterol), so the ratio is not changed.

Third, cholesterol is not usually the *root cause* of clogged up arteries—it's actually *inflammation*. Cholesterol simply shows up at the sight of inflammation and becomes the wrong focus instead of controlling inflammation.

These so-called "risk factors" all have poor diet, obesity, smoking, and excessive alcohol in common. Each can cause inflammation in the body—*that's* why they are risk factors. The cholesterol is actually the "good guy" that simply shows up at the site of inflammation to help reduce it. It's like firefighters trying to put out a fire; because they are at the fire doesn't make them "the bad guys" any more than cholesterol showing up to dampen the inflammation is bad.

In fact, the cholesterol-lowering prescription drug known as statins *causes* inflammation and robs the body of a very vital antioxidant called CoQ10, lowering the body's immune function. It makes no sense to prescribe something that causes inflammation to combat something that overcomes inflammation, but that is what is done. All. The. Time.

Now, I am not saying you are not at risk of heart disease based on this information alone, nor am I saying you don't need your medications any longer. I am merely trying to enlighten you to the truth about cholesterol. Don't be so quick to listen to what the drug companies are trying to tell you. Learn what your CRF is and make wise decisions based on the whole picture and not just a part of it.

To determine that most important number, the CRF, take your total cholesterol and divide your HDL into it; this will give you the Total:HDL ratio. You should have 3.0 or less for a healthy CRF, keeping in mind this is only one indicator that you are *not* at risk for heart disease. For example, let's say your total cholesterol is 300. You may be concerned or were told you are going to have a heart attack, and you need to be on medications NOW! Not so fast: let's look at the whole picture. In this example, we'll say your HDL is 100, which by the way is not unusual. My HDL is almost always over 100 and I will humbly admit I am not always the perfect specimen of health. If we do the above math, 300/100 results in 3.0, because your "good" cholesterol is high to begin with, but this is hardly ever taken into consideration. If you are viewing your cholesterol panel to see if you are at risk of heart disease, the most important number should be your CRF, not the Total or LDL.

In truth, a better test to determine your coronary risk where cholesterol is concerned is called a VAP test, which measures the *par-*

ticle sizes of the cholesterol molecules. Large particles cannot get into the blood vessels as smaller particles can. Before starting cholesterol medications simply because the drug companies say you need to ask your doctor to run a VAP test first. This is a relatively inexpensive test too, so even if your insurance doesn't cover it, pay cash for it and have it done. It is far better to do this before being put on a drug (for the rest of your life, no doubt) that causes inflammation, robs your body of vital immune-boosting nutrients like CoQ10, and is very toxic to your liver.

Also keep in mind that your cholesterol picture is only *one* risk factor in regard to your cardiovascular health; as mentioned others are obesity, smoking, diabetes, and family history of cardiovascular disease.

Another very important point about cholesterol is we actually *need* it. More times than there should have been, I had patients who had too low cholesterol and the medical doctors didn't think there was anything wrong with that. On a typical blood panel, the reference range for cholesterol is between 100-200. Looking at this reference range from a wholistic/wellness approach, it is 140-200, and I actually don't like to see a person's cholesterol below 170. If the cholesterol level is below 140, there may be neoplastic activity going on (i.e., cancer). Our immune system also needs cholesterol, as do most of our hormones, in order to be formed. Too often I see male patients with low cholesterol driven down by cholesterol medications, who are also on testosterone shots. Of course, their testosterone is going to be low when they don't have enough cholesterol!

I once had a patient who knew I practiced functional medicine but was only seeing me for chiropractic care; he preferred to go to the medical doctor for his "health." He shared with me that he was on cholesterol medications and that his TOTAL cholesterol was 87.

Some labs list their "normal" reference for cholesterol as "0-200." This would mean if a person had "0" cholesterol, or in this patient's case "87," it would never flag as too low. In the functional medicine world, if we see a total cholesterol below 140 it is considered an "ominous sign." This same patient also told me that he was receiving prescription testosterone shots. What would happen if he simply stopped taking cholesterol medications? His total cholesterol could possibly rise back up into the healthy range and he might not need the testosterone shots once his body had enough cholesterol to make hormones again. Even worse, if by not being concerned about too low cholesterol based on the range used by this particular lab, something very serious was going on with his health and he would never even know it until it was too late.

Contrary to what you might hear, high cholesterol is not because of too much dietary fat. It's because of diet and other life stressors causing inflammation in the body. I have already talked about an inflammatory diet vs. a non-inflammatory diet. If you want to lower your cholesterol, avoid inflammatory foods and eat non-inflammatory foods, and reduce stress.

One last point: When I view a new patient's cholesterol numbers and they are out of reference range—whether high OR low—the first place I start is the liver. The majority of the body's cholesterol is made in the liver, and it is quite possible a fatty, congested liver is the problem as opposed to cholesterol. One solution is to start with a liver detox.

The Truth about Thyroid and Iodine Testing

I meet so many people who either tell me they have hypothyroid, or they have all the symptoms of low thyroid but are told their blood work comes back normal. I am always leery of both of these diagnoses. In addition to being almost certain a comprehensive thyroid panel was not run, I also believe a major component of the whole thyroid picture was probably overlooked—the level of iodine in a person's body.

Every cell in the body needs iodine. The thyroid, breast tissue, uterus, ovaries, and testicles all need a heavy saturation of iodine, but most people are actually deficient in it. Polycystic Ovarian Syndrome (PCOS), cystic breasts, and uterine cysts could possibly be due to iodine deficiency. Instead of checking this first, major surgery removing the ovaries and/or uterus (i.e., hysterectomy) is performed. Alternatively, some women are put on a birth control pill to address the PCOS. This pill never allows the body to have a menstrual cycle and this is not normal. It also only addresses the symptoms and does not get to the root cause of the problem, which can actually cause more issues. These solutions send a woman down the path of a whole cascade of other health problems.

Iodine is needed for the uptake of the thyroid hormone in the body. Traditional medicine quite often just looks at the thyroid stimulating hormone (TSH), which is an anterior pituitary hormone and not really a thyroid hormone, and proceeds to tell the patient they have hypothyroidism; immediately thyroid medications are prescribed. In fact, the patient could be deficient in iodine instead and maybe not hypothyroid at all. Without testing the T4 and T3 markers, as well as other important thyroid markers, there would be no way to know for sure.

Iodine is a trace mineral. Chlorine, fluoride, and bromine are also trace minerals, but these elements are usually more abundant in the body than iodine is. They act like the "bullies on the block" in the body. Every cell has a special binding site on it that matches up perfectly to iodine, which allows the iodine to get into the cell. The binding site is like a lock and iodine is the key. Chlorine, fluoride, and bromine can also fit in the binding site, blocking iodine from getting in. People consume way too much chlorine and fluoride (from drinking water and toothpaste) and bromine (found in baked goods and packaged and processed foods). Even with a filter on your drinking water, unless you have a filter on your shower head as well, these minerals are getting into your skin and into your lungs (through the steam from the shower). If you're on well water, you are probably still getting these trace minerals from restaurants, convenience stores, and drive-through windows. We can also be deficient by simply not taking in enough iodine—but bleached-out table salt is not the place to get it.

There is a test called a "24-Hour Urine Test" that can measure the level of iodine as well as the other elements in your body. For this test, all of a patient's urine is caught and saved for a 24-hour period. A sampling of this urine is then sent off to a specialty lab where the level of each of these elements is tested. From these results an iodine deficiency can be determined as well as how much supplementation is needed. A few words of caution are warranted. If you do not know whether you are deficient in iodine, do *not* take iodine supplements in any measures larger than *micrograms* (mcg). Also, there are different schools of thought on whether patients with Hashimoto's thyroiditis (an autoimmune thyroid condition) should take any iodine (deficient or not). I encourage you to find a functional medicine doc you trust and pursue their protocol as advised.

Speaking of Hashimoto's, the lab work to rule this out is often not done. The TSH numbers and/or the T3 and T4 are *maybe* run, and if they are high and/or low, you are diagnosed with hypothyroid and put on thyroid medications for the rest of your life. If you are not tested for the thyroid antibodies to rule out Hashimoto's, you may never know if you have an autoimmune condition instead of a thyroid imbalance. If you have Hashimoto's, you are dealing with an *immune* issue, *not* a thyroid problem; these are two very different things and are addressed very differently when treated naturally.

In my experience, thyroid imbalances are typically secondary to another underlying root cause. Some of these primary root causes can be an anterior pituitary imbalance, adrenals that are out of balance, iodine deficiency, digestive and sugar imbalances, and immune imbalance. If you suspect you have thyroid problems, please be sure to address all of these other areas first before starting on a thyroid medication. Remember, medications do not "fix" the problem; they merely address the symptoms, and at best, manipulate your blood numbers back into reference range. Just because numbers change—whether they be thyroid, cholesterol, blood sugar, or anything else—it does not mean the problem has been fixed. If that were the case, you should be able to come off of your medications once the numbers are "normal," but that hardly ever happens.

I encourage you again to start looking at your health as whole—mental, emotional, physical, and spiritual. Your health IS in your control, working toward bringing your body back to good health using natural approaches. Look for a natural healthcare practitioner who will run a 24-hour urine iodine test for you if you suspect you have thyroid problems or have been told you need to go on medications.

I hope this has opened your eyes to the bigger picture about the truth in thyroid testing.

Comprehensive Digestive Stool Analysis (CDSA)

When I first started my functional medicine practice, I learned the many kinds of specialty lab testing that conventional medicine does not take the time to do. One, because they literally don't have time to do it. Two, it's not within their philosophy of practice. Three, they are not taught about it (because this is not within the pharmaceutical industry's scope, and that's who educates them). Four, insurance won't pay for it.

As much as was reasonable, I would be my own "guinea pig" and run these various specialty tests on myself, including a Comprehensive Digestive Stool Analysis test (CDSA).

You may recall I talked about the digestive system being one of the most important systems in our body. The CDSA is an excellent test to determine a starting point for the integrity level of the digestive system. This test is a little more expensive as far as specialty lab testing goes, so if you and your practitioner think your digestive system is in pretty good shape and maybe just needs some supplemental support, then perhaps start there. But if you are experiencing symptoms directly related to your digestion or altered immune function, I highly encourage you to pursue this test. It reveals a wealth of information about the state of your overall health.

It will assess the levels of good and bad bacteria, good and bad levels of yeast, the presence of any parasites (more Americans have parasites than realize it!), gut intolerances to certain foods, the absorption capabilities of the gut (whether nutrients are being reabsorbed or proteins are sneaking in where they don't belong), and so much more.

This test is truly worth its value and a great place to start when assessing one's health.

Neurotransmitter Testing

I know too many people who have been diagnosed for years as being depressed, yet they've *never* had a neurotransmitter test run. They have been diagnosed subjectively based on symptoms. Each time they go back to the doctor, their medications get adjusted based on the same method—that is, how the patient has been "feeling" (which by the way is usually lousy, more so because of the medications than the chemical imbalance). This to me is one of the greatest atrocities of conventional medicine, and I feel there are many.

This is such a serious diagnosis that the cost of a vital neurotransmitter test should not even be questioned by the insurance companies; in essence it is putting that price on a life. I will even go so far as suggesting that in some cases emotional issues that are not addressed from the root can lead to a very slippery slope: drug addiction, leading to greater mental health problems, which then leads to poverty, broken families, homelessness, and at times criminal records.

Think back to our discussion of trauma and addiction. Anxiety and depression certainly were two of the many symptoms you could expect to find associated with addiction, trauma, *and* diet. How valuable would this test be? Let me tell you about it, so you can answer with an educated decision.

Neurotransmitters are our brain hormones or brain chemicals, particularly, epinephrine, norepinephrine, dopamine, serotonin, GABA, and acetylcholine as well as hormones like leptin and ghrelin (the brain chemicals that regulate our appetite) and melatonin, the chemical that regulates our sleep.

These brain chemicals have a direct influence on our reproductive hormones like estrogen, testosterone, and progesterone, which in turn influence our brain chemicals. They also communicate with the thyroid hormone. The health conditions associated with these are numerous.

This test can first reveal the current levels of each neurotransmitter and hormone. From there we can assess which ones are too high and too low and determine the support needed accordingly—ideally from a wholistic natural approach. Yet even if one decided to take mood-altering pharmaceutical medications, it would be just as important, if not more so, to test these levels regularly rather than simply going by how someone "feels." After all, when someone is anxious or depressed, it could be a safe assumption their assessment would naturally be skewed by what was really going on in the body. With the ultimate goal being the patient feeling better, regular testing of these vital hormones is a far better approach than just "guessing."

In my opinion, this is an extremely vital and probably the most overlooked test throughout the psychology world. This is a test within the scope of practice for a functional medicine doctor, especially one who specifically addresses these heart-rending health issues.

Call to Action: I recommend starting with a cholesterol panel, which is relatively simple and one lab test most of us probably have had at some time in the past. Rather than viewing it from the conventional approach, however, calculate your coronary risk factor (CRF) by taking your total cholesterol number and dividing your HDL into it. You will want to see 3.0 or less. Armed with this knowledge now, you can determine if you really have "high cholesterol." If you are on cholesterol medications and your CRF is 3.0 or less, you should discuss with your practitioner whether you really need to be on those medications. Recall the risk factors of being on cholesterol medications include their toxic effects on the liver and the depletion of the vital antioxidant CoQ10, just to name a few.

If you are on cholesterol medications simply based on your total cholesterol and/or your LDL being high or if your CRF number is greater than 3.0, then I suggest having a VAP test run to learn the particle sizes of the cholesterol. It is quite common for some people who have what looks like a "normal" cholesterol reading to have a positive VAP test, while others who have what looks like high cholesterol have a negative or "good" VAP test.

If you are on thyroid medications based on the very basic thyroid labs, go back to the doctor who has you on the medications and insist on having a complete and comprehensive thyroid panel including but not limited to the thyroid antibodies TPO and TGB. If they will not do this for you, find yourself another practitioner—ideally a functional medicine doc who will assess your thyroid completely and accurately.

If you are on antidepressants and/or anxiety medications, I highly encourage you to seek out a functional medicine doctor who will order a neurotransmitter test for you.

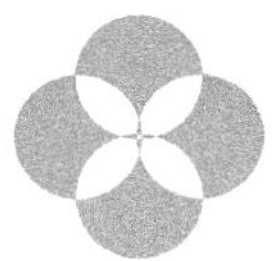

Conclusion

"And now, a word to you who are elders in the churches. I, too, am an elder and a witness to the sufferings of Christ. And I, too, will share in his glory when he is revealed to the whole world. As a fellow elder, I appeal to you: Care for the flock that God has entrusted to you. Watch over it willingly, not grudgingly—not for what you will get out of it, but because you are eager to serve God. Don't lord it over the people assigned to your care, but lead them by your own good example. And when the Great Shepherd appears, you will receive a crown of never-ending glory and honor. "

—1 Peter 5:1-4 NLT

There you have it—the truth about wellness. You can now take what you started off knowing about health and wellness back off the shelf where you placed it before reading this book and ask yourself which paradigm do you now want to follow?

This information certainly is not all inclusive, nor is it intended to be. I believe new truths will continue to present themselves every day. In fact, as of the publication of this book as well as its companion online video course, the tide is already beginning to shift where our government here in the United States is concerned. Robert F. Kennedy Jr. (RFK Jr.) is now the Secretary of the Department of Health and Human Resources (HHS), and he is already making tremendous strides towards righting the ship, and putting health back on its proper course. I remain hopeful that we will finally see the health of our nation here in America be restored–especially as it pertains to children and our next generation. As I was beginning to hear the heart of RFK Jr., as well as those he chose for his under-secretaries in the various departments under HHS, I felt they had already read this book–they are "singing my song!"

Hopefully this information will get you started by putting your feet on a new wholistic path with your eyes wide open—onto the path of health and healing instead of simply and blindly riding the rails of destruction and disease. Hopefully there is now the light of belief and confidence in your eyes, and in your heart knowing your health IS in your control and you are educated, empowered, and ready to embark on the journey of FREEDOM that exists for all of us! Any step in "restoring your body back to good health" is a step in the right direction, and it can simply start with one small step at a time.

My prayer is that as you pursue these truths, you are now able to go out and fulfill your purpose with certainty and passion—healthy and whole—and share these messages of truth with others so that they can do the same and the entire world can be a healthier place to live!

Blessings & Health,
Dr. Jackie McKool

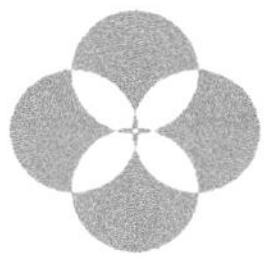

APPENDIX A

Suggested Reading and Resources

When I sat down to write up my suggested reading list, I truly just wanted to take a picture of all of my bookshelves (yes, plural) and include it in this Appendix. There are so many great resources out there and I drew from so many over the years. I tried to include those that are my favorites and those I referenced in this book. This list represents a cross-section of books on the topics I covered here—again, certainly not all inclusive but a great place to start. Many of these authors also have websites, so I highly suggest checking them out as well.

Books

What to Say When You Talk to Yourself, by Shad Helmstetter, Ph.D.

True Confessions of an Rx Drug Pusher by Gwen Olsen

Death by Medicine by Gary Null, Ph.D.

Food & Behavior, A Natural Connection by Barbara Reed Stitt

Why is My Brain Not Working by Datis Kharrazian, DHSc., D.C., M.S.

No More Dirty Looks by Siobhan O'Connor & Alexandra Spunt

How to Hear God's Voice by Mark Virkler

Sick & Tired? Reclaim Your Inner Terrain by Dr. Robert Young

The pH Miracle, Balance Your Diet, Reclaim Your Health by Dr. Robert Young

Hope, Medicine & Healing by Francisco Contreras, M.D. & Daniel E. Kennedy, M.C.

Beyond Gluten Intolerance by Karen Masterson Koch, C.N.

The Miracle of Magnesium by Dr. Carolyn Dean

The Healing Revolution by Dr. Frank King

Why Stomach Acid is Good for You by Jonathan V. Wright, M.D. & Lane Lenard, Ph.D.

Salt Your Way to Health by David Brownstein, M.D.

Overcoming Thyroid Disorders by David Brownstein, M.D.

MycoMedicinals, An Informational Treatise on Mushrooms by Paul Stamets

Your Body's Many Cries for Water by F. Batmanghelidj, M.D.

Gut Solutions by Brenda Watson, N.D.

Back to Eden by Jethro Kloss

Salt, Sugar, Fat by Michael Moss

Cancer – Step Outside the Box by Ty Bollinger

The Overspent American, Why We Want What We Don't Have by Juliet B. Schor

The Overworked American, the Unexpected Decline of Leisure by Juliet B. Schor

Raw Food & Alkalizing Recipe Books

Raw Food, A Complete Guide for Every Meal of the Day by Erica Palmcrantz and

Irmelda Lilja

The Hallelujah Diet, Experience the Optimal Health You Were Meant to Have by

George Malkmus

Everyday Raw by Matthew Kenney

Ani's Raw Food Essentials by Ani Phyo

Alkaline Diet Recipe Book (Volume I & II) by Ross Bridgeford

Businesses/Organizations

Biotics Detox -- https://us.fullscript.com/welcome/jmckool

Renew Life Liver Detox --

https://www.betteryourhealth.com/renewlife/product/liver-detox

Prescription Drug Classifications -- https://americanaddictioncenters.org/prescription-drugs/classifications

Hulda Clark's gallbladder flush -- at https://drclark.net/en-us/cleanses/liver-cleanse-page/liver-cleanse-recipe2

Mg12 Magnesium – www.mg12.com

Oasis of Hope Cancer Treatment Center – https://www.oasisofhope.com/

Gaia Herbs Farm - https://www.gaiaherbs.com/pages/our-farm

Frontier Co-op - https://www.frontiercoop.com/

Alliance for Natural Health - https://anh-usa.org/

Communion With God Ministries, at www.cwgministries.org

Dave Ramsey, Financial Peace University, www.ramseysolutions.com

Cleansing Stream, www.cleansingstream.org

Healing Rooms Ministries, www.healingrooms.com

Resources to find Wholistic Practitioners

The American Chiropractic Association's Council on Diagnosis and Internal Disorders (CDID) https://aca-cdid.com/

The Chiropractic Board of Clinical Nutrition

https://www.cbcn.us/

The American Chiropractic Association Council on Nutrition

https://www.councilonnutrition.com/

The American Clinical Board of Nutrition (ACBN)

https://www.acbn.org/

American Nutrition Association

https://theana.org/

The Institute for Functional Medicine

https://www.ifm.org/find-a-practitioner/

Functional Medicine University

https://www.functionalmedicineuniversity.com/public/find-Functional-Medicine-Clinicians.cfm

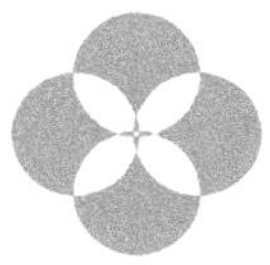

APPENDIX B

How to Hear God's Voice

by Dr. Mark Virkler

She had done it again! Instead of coming straight home from school like she was supposed to, she had gone to her friend's house. Without permission. Without our knowledge. Without doing her chores.

With a ministering household that included remnants of three struggling families plus our own toddler and newborn, my wife simply couldn't handle all the work on her own. Everyone had to pull their own weight. Everyone had age-appropriate tasks they were expected to complete. At fourteen, Rachel and her younger brother were living with us while her parents tried to overcome lifestyle patterns that had resulted in the children running away to escape the dysfunction. I felt sorry for Rachel, but, honestly, my wife was my greatest concern.

Now Rachel had ditched her chores to spend time with her friends. It wasn't the first time, but if I had anything to say about it, it would be the last. I intended to lay down the law when she got home and make it very clear that if she was going to live under my roof, she would obey my rules.

But…she wasn't home yet. And I had recently been learning to hear God's voice more clearly. Maybe I should try to see if I could hear anything from Him about the situation. Maybe He could give me a way to get her to do what she was supposed to (i.e. what I wanted her to do). So I went to my office and reviewed what the Lord had been teaching me from Habakkuk 2:1,2: "I will stand on my guard post and station myself on the rampart; And I will keep watch to see what He will speak to me…Then the Lord answered me and said, 'Record the vision….'"

Habakkuk said, "I will stand on my guard post..." (Hab. 2:1). The first key to hearing God's voice is to go to a quiet place and still our own thoughts and emotions. Psalm 46:10 encourages us to be still, let go, cease striving, and know that He is God. In Psalm 37:7 we are called to "be still before the Lord and wait patiently for Him." There is a deep inner knowing in our spirits that each of us can experience when we quiet our flesh and our minds. Practicing the art of biblical meditation helps silence the outer noise and distractions clamoring for our attention.

I didn't have a guard post, but I did have an office, so I went there to quiet my temper and my mind. Loving God through a quiet worship song is one very effective way to become still. In 2 Kings 3, Elisha needed a word from the Lord, so he said, "Bring me a minstrel," and as the minstrel played, the Lord spoke. I have found that playing a worship song on my autoharp is the quickest way for me to come to stillness. I need to choose my song carefully; boisterous songs of praise do not bring me to stillness, but rather gentle songs that express my love and worship. And it isn't enough just to sing the song into the cosmos—I come into the Lord's presence most quickly and easily when I use my godly imagination to see the truth that He is right here with me and I sing my songs to Him, personally.

"I will keep watch to see," said the prophet. To receive the pure word of God, it is very important that my heart be properly focused as I become still, because my focus is the source of the intuitive flow. If I fix my eyes upon Jesus (Heb. 12:2), the intuitive flow comes from Jesus. But if I fix my gaze upon some desire of my heart, the intuitive flow comes out of that desire. To have a pure flow I must become still and carefully fix my eyes upon Jesus. Quietly worshiping the King and receiving out of the stillness that follows quite easily accomplishes this.

So, I used the second key to hearing God's voice: As you pray, fix the eyes of your heart upon Jesus, seeing in the Spirit the dreams and visions of Almighty God. Habakkuk was actually looking for vision as he prayed. He opened the eyes of his heart and looked into the spirit world to see what God wanted to show him.

God has always spoken through dreams and visions, and He specifically said that they would come to those upon whom the Holy Spirit is poured out (Acts 2:1-4, 17).

Being a logical, rational person, observable facts that could be verified by my physical senses were the foundations of my life, including my spiritual life. I had never thought of opening the eyes of my heart and looking for vision. However, I have come to believe that this is exactly what God wants me to do. He gave me eyes in my heart to see in the spirit the vision and movement of Almighty God.

There is an active spirit world all around us, full of angels, demons, the Holy Spirit, the omnipresent Father, and His omnipresent Son, Jesus. The only reasons for me not to see this reality are unbelief or lack of knowledge.

In his sermon in Acts 2:25, Peter refers to King David's statement: "I saw the Lord always in my presence; for He is at my right hand, so that I will not be shaken." The original psalm makes it clear that this was a decision of David's, not a constant supernatural visitation: "I have set (literally, I have placed) the Lord continually before me; because He is at my right hand, I will not be shaken" (Ps.16:8). Because David knew that the Lord was always with him, he determined in his spirit to see that truth with the eyes of his heart as he went through life, knowing that this would keep his faith strong.

In order to see, we must look. Daniel saw a vision in his mind and said, "I was looking...I kept looking...I kept looking" (Dan. 7:2, 9, 13). As I pray, I look for Jesus, and I watch as He speaks to me, doing and saying the things that are in His heart. Many Christians will find that if they only look, they will see. Jesus is Emmanuel, God with us (Matt. 1:23). It is as simple as that. You can see Christ present with you because Christ is present with you. In fact, the vision may come so easily that you will be tempted to reject it, thinking that it is just you. But if you persist in recording these visions, your doubt will soon be overcome by faith as you recognize that the content of them could only be birthed in Almighty God.

Jesus demonstrated the ability of living out of constant contact with God, declaring that He did nothing on His own initiative, but only what He saw the Father doing, and heard the Father saying (Jn. 5:19,20,30). What an incredible way to live!

Is it possible for us to live out of divine initiative as Jesus did? Yes! We must simply fix our eyes upon Jesus. The veil has been torn, giving access into the immediate presence of God, and He calls us to draw near (Lk. 23:45; Heb. 10:19-22). "I pray that the eyes of your heart will be enlightened…."

When I had quieted my heart enough that I was able to picture Jesus without the distractions of my own ideas and plans, I was able to "keep watch to see what He will speak to me." I wrote down my question: "Lord, what should I do about Rachel?"

Immediately the thought came to me, "She is insecure." Well, that certainly wasn't my thought! Her behavior looked like rebellion to me, not insecurity.

But like Habakkuk, I was coming to know the sound of God speaking to me (Hab. 2:2). Elijah described it as a still, small voice (I Kings 19:12). I had previously listened for an inner audible voice, and God does speak that way at times. However, I have found that usually, God's voice comes as spontaneous thoughts, visions, feelings, or impressions.

For example, haven't you been driving down the road and had a thought come to you to pray for a certain person? Didn't you believe it was God telling you to pray? What did God's voice sound like? Was it an audible voice, or was it a spontaneous thought that lit upon your mind?

Experience indicates that we perceive spirit-level communication as spontaneous thoughts, impressions and visions, and Scripture confirms this in many ways. For example, one definition of paga, a Hebrew word for intercession, is "a chance encounter or an accidental intersecting." When God lays people on our hearts, He does it through paga, a chance-encounter thought "accidentally" intersecting our minds.

So, the third key to hearing God's voice is recognizing that God's voice in your heart often sounds like a flow of spontaneous thoughts. Therefore, when I want to hear from God, I tune to chance-encounter or spontaneous thoughts.

Finally, God told Habakkuk to record the vision (Hab. 2:2). This was not an isolated command. The Scriptures record many examples of individual's prayers and God's replies, such as the Psalms, many of the prophets, and Revelation. I have found that obeying this final principle amplified my confidence in my ability to hear God's voice so that I could finally make living out of His initiatives a way of life. The fourth key, two-way journaling or the writing out of your prayers and God's answers, brings great freedom in hearing God's voice.

I have found two-way journaling to be a fabulous catalyst for clearly discerning God's inner, spontaneous flow, because as I journal, I am able to write in faith for long periods of time, simply believing it is God. I know that what I believe I have received from God must be tested. However, testing involves doubt and doubt blocks divine communication, so I do not want to test while I am trying to receive. (See James 1:5-8.) With journaling, I can receive in faith, knowing that when the flow has ended, I can test and examine it carefully.

So, I wrote down what I believed He had said: "She is insecure."

But the Lord wasn't done. I continued to write the spontaneous thoughts that came to me: "Love her unconditionally. She is flesh of your flesh and bone of your bone."

My mind immediately objected: She is not flesh of my flesh. She is not related to me at all—she is a foster child, just living in my home temporarily. It was definitely time to test this "word from the Lord"!

There are three possible sources of thoughts in our minds: ourselves, Satan and the Holy Spirit. It was obvious that the words in my journal did not come from my own mind—I certainly didn't see her as insecure or the flesh of my flesh. And I sincerely doubted that Satan would encourage me to love anyone unconditionally!

Okay, it was starting to look like I might have actually received counsel from the Lord. It was consistent with the names and character of God as revealed in the Scripture, and totally contrary to the names and character of the enemy. So that meant that I was hearing from the Lord, and He wanted me to see the situation in a different light. Rachel was my daughter—part of my family not by blood but by the hand of God Himself. The chaos of her birth home had created deep insecurity about her worthiness to be loved by anyone, including me and including God. Only the unconditional love of the Lord expressed through an imperfect human would reach her heart.

But there was still one more test I needed to perform before I would have absolute confidence that this was truly God's word to me: I needed confirmation from someone else whose spiritual discernment I trusted. So, I went to my wife and shared what I had received. I knew if I could get her validation, especially since she was the one most wronged in the situation, then I could say, at least to myself, "Thus saith the Lord."

Needless to say, Patti immediately and without question confirmed that the Lord had spoken to me. My entire planned lecture was forgotten. I returned to my office anxious to hear more. As the Lord planted a new, supernatural love for Rachel within me, He showed me what to say and how to say it to not only address the current issue of household responsibility, but the deeper issues of love and acceptance and worthiness.

Rachel and her brother remained as part of our family for another two years, giving us many opportunities to demonstrate and teach about the Father's love, planting spiritual seeds in thirsty soil. We weren't perfect and we didn't solve all of her issues, but because I had learned to listen to the Lord, we were able to avoid creating more brokenness and separation.

The four simple keys that the Lord showed me from Habakkuk have been used by people of all ages, from four to a hundred and four, from every continent, culture and denomination, to break through into intimate two-way conversations with their loving Father and dearest Friend. Omitting any one of the keys will prevent you from receiving all He wants to say to you. The order of the keys is not important, just that you use them all. Embracing all four, by faith, can change your life. Simply quiet yourself down, tune to spontaneity, look for vision, and journal.

He is waiting to meet you there.

You will be amazed when you journal! Doubt may hinder you at first, but throw it off, reminding yourself that it is a biblical concept, and that God is present, speaking to His children. Relax. When we cease our labors and enter His rest, God is free to flow (Heb. 4:10).

Why not try it for yourself, right now? Sit back comfortably, take out your pen and paper, and smile. Turn your attention toward the Lord in praise and worship, seeking His face. Many people have found the music and visionary prayer called "A Stroll Along the Sea of Galilee" helpful in getting them started. You can listen to it and download it for free at www.CWGMinistries.org/Galilee.

After you write your question to Him, become still, fixing your gaze on Jesus. You will suddenly have a very good thought. Don't doubt it; simply write it down. Later, as you read your journaling, you, too, will be blessed to discover that you are indeed dialoguing with God. If you wonder if it is really the Lord speaking to you, share it with your spouse or a friend. Their input will encourage your faith and strengthen your commitment to spend time getting to know the Lover of your soul more intimately than you ever dreamed possible.

Is It Really God?

Five ways to be sure what you're hearing is from Him:

1) Test the Origin (1 Jn. 4:1)

   Thoughts from our own minds are progressive, with one thought leading to the next, however tangentially. Thoughts from the spirit world are spontaneous. The Hebrew word for true prophecy is *naba*, which literally means to bubble up, whereas false prophecy is *ziyd* meaning to boil up. True words from the Lord will bubble up from our innermost being; we don't need to cook them up ourselves.

2) Compare It to Biblical Principles

   God will never say something to you personally which is contrary to His universal revelation as expressed in the Scriptures. If the Bible clearly states that something is a sin, no amount of journaling can make it right. Much of what you journal about will not be specifically addressed in the Bible, however, so an understanding of biblical principles is also needed.

3) Compare It to the Names and Character of God as Revealed in the Bible

Anything God says to you will be in harmony with His essential nature. Journaling will help you get to know God personally, but knowing what the Bible says about Him will help you discern what words are from Him. Make sure the tenor of your journaling lines up with the character of God as described in the names of the Father, Son and Holy Spirit.

4) Test the Fruit (Matt. 7:15-20)

   What effect does what you are hearing have on your soul and your spirit? Words from the Lord will quicken your faith and increase your love, peace and joy. They will stimulate a sense of humility within you as you become more aware of Who God is and who you are. On the other hand, any words you receive which cause you to fear or doubt, which bring you into confusion or anxiety, or which stroke.

   your ego (especially if you hear something that is "just for you alone—no one else is worthy") must be immediately rebuked and rejected as lies of the enemy.

5) Share It with Your Spiritual Counselors (Prov. 11:14)

   We are members of a Body! A cord of three strands is not easily broken and God's intention has always been for us to grow together. Nothing will increase your faith in your ability to hear from God like having it confirmed by two or three other people! Share it with your spouse, your parents, your friends, your elder, your group leader, even your grown children can be your sounding board. They don't need to be perfect or super-spiritual; they just need to love you, be committed to being available to you, have a solid biblical orientation, and most importantly, they must also willingly and easily receive counsel. Avoid the authoritarian who insists that because of their standing in the church or with God, they no longer need to listen to others. Find two or three people and let them confirm that you are hearing from God! The book 4 Keys to Hearing God's Voice is available at https://www.cwgministries.org/4keys.

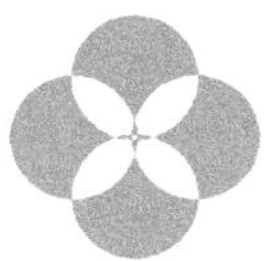

About the Author

Dr. Jackie McKool has been passionate about wholistic health and wellness since God delivered her in 1996 from an addiction to alcohol and the whole bar life. He pulled her out of the miry clay and set her feet on a new path—a wholistic path of health and healing. She believes with all her heart and soul that God has called her to speak, teach, and write with the purpose of glorifying Him.

Dr. McKool spent 10 years in the wholistic health and wellness field as a chiropractic physician in Charleston, South Carolina. She has her post-doctorate in Internal Disorders, which is similar to a doctor of natural medicine. Dr. McKool is one of less than 500 worldwide board-certified Chiropractic Internists with a focus on Internal Disorders. Upon moving to North Carolina, she worked in the natural products industry in several health food stores for three years.

Dr. Jackie has served as a trained minister for several Christian healing ministries, including Cleansing Stream founded by Pastor Jack Hayford, and the International Healing Rooms Ministries founded by Rev. Cal Pierce. She has also studied under Dr. Mark Virkler, founder of Christian Leadership University and Communion with God Ministries. Dr. Virkler is also the author of "4 Keys to Hearing God's Voice."

In addition to wholistic health and wellness, Dr. Jackie loves being in God's creation outdoors. She claims she was "born to be outside!" She loves jogging, hiking, biking, kayaking, and most of all backpacking. At the age of 65, she recently completed her 11-year journey of backpacking the Appalachian Trail (AT), a 2,200-mile-long foot trail by summiting Mt. Katahdin on August 11th, 2024. Look for her next book that is already brewing pertaining to her adventures on the AT!

She lives in western North Carolina with her two fur baby cats: KoKo and Sadie. To reach Dr. Jackie for speaking opportunities or to follow her blog posts she can be found:

On her website: **www.jackiemckool.com**
By email: **jackie@jackiemckool.com**
or Facebook: **www.facebook.com/drjackiemckool**

Want more? Scan the QR code below and gain VIP access to Jackie's latest news, inspiring resources, and exclusive updates!

www.ingramcontent.com/pod-product-compliance
Lightning Source LLC
Chambersburg PA
CBHW062117020426
42335CB00013B/1000
9781965401736